Getting There

Getting There

Navigating Holistic Care

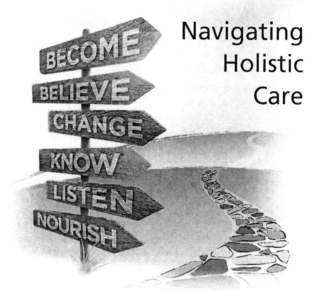

Jean Bennett

I dedicate this book to my brother. Even though he probably doesn't know it, he's my daily inspiration to not sweat the small stuff, but instead, find its humor. You, my dear brother, are my driving force to learn more. Your ability to say, "Yes," every day, inspires us all and sends ripples of encouraging energy throughout the universe. This I know. I love you.

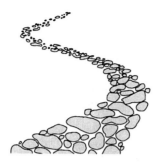

CONTENTS

Acknowledgements xi
Prologue xiii

PART I: JESSIE'S STORY
1   Introduction to the Problem 3
    Stress 4
2   Coming up with a Plan 7
    Perceptions 8
    Body Signs 9
    More about Body Structure and Mechanics 11
    Fibromyalgia Tolerance Levels 13
    Homework 14
    Chest Breathing 17
    Making a Plan 19
3   Getting Started 21
    Religions 24
    Strengthening Intent 26
    Digestion and Enzymes 29
    Wheat, Sugar and GMOs 31

How the Stomach Works 34

More About Nutrition 36

Why Holistic Health Care Is So Hard 40

Grounding 42

The Nervous System—SNS and PSNS 43

Conscious and Subconscious 45

4 The Grind 51

Cleanup Crew 52

Energy and Why Emotions Matter 54

Healing Crises 58

What We Say Matters 64

Pesky Energy, and Spirits 66

Energy Vampires 71

About Antidepressants 73

Different from Counseling 75

5 Don't Give Up 77

Yin and Yang 81

Deep Core Beliefs 83

Following the Threads—The Whys and the Yea-buts 85

Protection 90

6 The Roller Coaster 93

Intuition—Guides, Universal Energy, or Imagination 99

Owning Your Power 107

Emotional House of Cards 109

Be the Observer 119

7 Finally, Relief! 121

8 Summary 129

PART II: GETTING THERE—BEYOND WELLNESS

9 Helping More Than Yourself 137

The Balance of Wellness 138

Both Sides of the Control Coin 145

10 Changing Beliefs 151
    Releasing the Negative 151
    Creating the Positive 157

PART III: WHAT TO DO IF

11 Why, What, How, and Who 163
12 If You have a Chronic or Serious Issue 169
13 If You are Helping Someone Else 177
14 If You are a Holistic Practitioner 181
15 If You are an Allopathic Doctor 185
16 If You are in Medical Insurance,
    Education, or Regulation 191

Epilogue 197
Appendix A: Body Babble 205
Reference: Recommended Books 225
About the Author 231

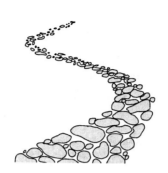

ACKNOWLEDGEMENTS

First and foremost, I'd like to thank Jessie for her courage in sharing her very personal story. Without her and her desire to help others, I suspect this book would never have been written. The proof reading for accuracy was especially difficult for her because she had to revisit some still raw moments, but she did it anyway, even though she had no obligation to do so…just another indicator of her big heart. Thank you Jessie, from the depths of my soul, for inspiring our readers and for helping me to educate them about how they can help themselves.

No book is complete without great editors, and I had several who each brought a different perspective to round out the explanations and information so Jessie and I could reach more people. My heartfelt thanks to Barbara Barber, Mario Cerasuolo, Deb Disbrow, Chris Linsner-Cartwright, and The Zebra Ink. Also, my very special thanks go to my treasured friends Barbara and Mario, and to my mom, Joan Bennett, for our many in depth conversations that helped pull together the more complex ideas and critical points. Without all of you, our readers would probably not make it past the prologue.

Those of us working with energy need someone who is not afraid to get in the trenches with us. The one who will tell you when you're thinking has got the best of you, and pull you back; who will encourage your wacky ideas that push your growth; and who has your back and allows you to have theirs. Barbara is all of this for me and more. I would not be as far as I am in this career if not for her encouragement, her friendship, and her willingness to call me on my stuff. Much, much love and gratitude to you, Barbara, my dear friend and colleague.

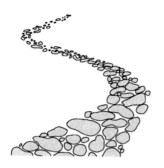

PROLOGUE

I was a successful business executive in the corporate world. It was great fun whisking around the globe, having the CEOs' assistants say, "I have a limo waiting to take you to the airport, Ms. Bennett." The money was good and I was learning tons about many different companies; their management styles; what worked; and what didn't. I even ended up owning my own company in the software arena of that world. Some would say life was grand and I was living the ultimate dream.

I hated it. I couldn't breathe. It was killing me. I wasn't ready to die yet.

I was fortunate to be able to sell the company and get out of the situation I was sure to cause my death within a fleeting time. I wanted to meet my grandkids, so I got busy to get healthy again.

However, in the world I knew (and much to my surprise) there was no help. The stomach pains were only indigestion, so "Deal with it and take Tums." The bloating and cramps were only because I ate the wrong things, so "Stop eating them." The heart palpations, arrhythmia, and chest pains had no known cause, so "Wait and if it gets worse we can do something then." Not being able to breathe was all in my head, so "Take anti-anxiety pills." The chronic fatigue was because I was getting older, so "Get more sleep."

"Really! I can't function and this is all you have to offer!?" It was obvious by then that our medical system knew little about stress-related illnesses.

A few years before this time my sister and I went to a psychic fair for an afternoon of fun and finding out what all "those weird people" were about. I ended up volunteering for a reiki demonstration and when the woman's hand floated over my chest area her expression went into...*alarm face*. She was polite and said only, "There's a little something going on here," but I saw her face and took note that maybe there was something to this.

In my frustration with our medical system, this memory came flooding back. I rushed to my desk, hoping I still had her card as I rifled through the drawers. Yes! I still had it.

My first session was eye-opening and life-changing. I saw colors behind my eyelids that I had never seen before, and it felt like I had three glasses of wine. It opened up a whole new world to me that I hadn't known existed. None of my issues were gone in this first session (as I had secretly hoped) but it showed me that there really was something to this and I had to know more. My journey to the answers I needed had begun.

My travels took me through the history of our medical system and our extraordinarily ancient world. It took me to the old ways of healing and to new ways of applying them; to the inner being; to cosmic comprehension of time and space and other realities and dimensions; to the workings of cells; to quantum physics; and to the interdependency of all being one. But, most of all, it helped me become the "new me." With my shiny new toolbox, I was able to recognize and deal with my long-held deep core issues that were holding me back. "Getting there" for me took a couple of years, but inch by inch, I got my health back. The journey has not stopped, but instead has become a continuous procession of learning, loving, and living within the awesomeness of the physical and emotional world we call Earth.

This brings me to why I wrote this book. Our medical system is in transition from a basis in Newtonian physics to a basis in quantum physics. These two systems are complete opposites. Newtonian belief is "anything energetic is manifested from the physical," and quantum belief is "anything physical is manifested from the energetic." Energy medicine has been practiced in Eastern countries for over 5000 years, and it was proven through our scientific methods by Einstein in the early 1900's. It has since been labeled "quantum belief." (I guess it takes us a while to catch up.)

This is turning everything about our medical system on its head. There are those stuck in the old ways and those pushing hard for the new. There are antiquated systems and procedures, and there are totally uncharted territories for regulations and licensing. There are individuals in both camps screaming the illegitimacy of the other. Our accepted educational institutions are still teaching the old material while new classes are springing up everywhere to teach the new. In other words, IT'S CHAOS OUT THERE!

Even the names are confusing. There are many terms that may mean the same thing to different people, like "energetic medicine," quantum, eastern, holistic, alternative, or integrative care. So to keep things straight, I'll be using three terms:

1) **Allopathic medicine** refers to our standard medical system in the USA, which is based in the physical.

2) **Energy medicine** refers to the modalities of the eastern ways, which are based in the energetic.

3) **Holistic care** refers to the blend of both...our future health care system.

Do not get frustrated. Just understand that change brings chaos and differences of opinion. Your job is to make conscious choices about how to weed your way through it. And, THAT is what this book is about—helping you sort through the chaos while our world is making its transition to a fabulous new holistic care system that brings the skills of the Western physical ways together with the skills of the Eastern energetic ways. This transition is affecting the entire world—our health care, our economic systems, our governments, and our core beliefs and way of living. We all need to pitch in and help in this process by fixing our issues and staying healthy and happy. Helping you get to healthy and happy, from wherever you are starting from, is what this book is about.

"There" is defined by each goal you set, and it gets redefined as you get there. As used in this book, "there" is a malleable term that is different for everyone and changes for different times in your life. What "getting there" means depends on where you are. It may mean getting rid of a chronic issue or pain, getting a different job, finding peace of mind, or learning how to move forward with family dynamics. There is something in here for all problems and for all ages.

I introduce the tool sets through Jessie and her journey from pain to wellness. All of Jessie's story is true, although a few facts have been changed to protect Jessie's identity. I diverge often into educational tutorials to help you understand "the whys and the wherefores" and to give you a deeper comprehension.

There are three ways to read this book:

1) Read it start to finish as normal

2) Read Jessie's story first which is in italics

3) Read the education tutorials first which are in normal type.

You will learn ways in which your body and the universe talk to you through its babbling signs; how to listen; and what to do about it.

This symbol (✍) lets you know a tutorial about that subject will follow soon after. I have organized it so you can easily get back to information years later, so keep this book in your reference library because, if you are like the rest of us, you'll probably only retain a small portion of what you read. So, don't worry if it doesn't click in or resonate with you the first time around.

If you are the need-to-know-more type, there is a list of books for your exploring pleasure in the Reference section at the end. Their numbers are throughout the book to point you to further information.

As always, pick out what is right for you at the time and ignore the rest. Some of the information is right for you now, some may be right for you in a year or two, and some may not ever be right for you. My hope is to prompt you to take hold of the reins yourself, with full understanding that there are many ways, beyond our current medical system, to "getting there."

Happy reading! Wishing You Love, Light, and Laughter.

Jean Bennett, Energy Therapist, LMT

PART I
JESSIE'S STORY

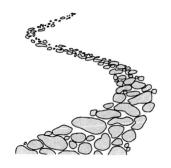

"So many difficulties in your life probably exist because the current data set you are operating from has not yet expanded to hold the burgeoning buoyancy of soluble solutions from beyond."

— Marilyn Gewacke, PhD —

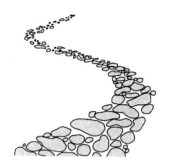

CHAPTER 1
Introduction to the Problem

Jessie's Story ☞

Jessie is a gal whose pain in her neck and shoulders was so bad it was changing her life, her mood, and her outlook on everything. When I first saw her in April she had been experiencing this pain on and off for three years, and this episode had been continuous since November... nearly six months. She was at her wits' end and had lost all hope of having her life back. She was looking at the rest of her years being filled with prescriptions, side effects and more debilitating pain.

Her doctors could find nothing physically wrong and had diagnosed her pain as fibromyalgia. They suggested seeing an orthopedic specialist and when he also, could do nothing for her, he told her to try massage to help with the symptoms. That is how Jessie ended up with me...I was the lucky one to get her call when she contacted our office of seven practitioners.

Jessie's Health History

My observation of Jesse upon first meeting her was that she was in incredibly good physical shape for her age of 70. She walked with normal length and quick strides; could bend and sit like a much younger person (she did not fall into a chair); she was at a good weight; and her breathing did not change as she climbed the stairs to my office. She also carried her shoulders up by her ears, which was an indicator of the amount of pain she was in.

Jessie's chief complaint was pain from the fibromyalgia, which was primarily in her lower neck to the back of her skull and often wrapping around to the clavicle area in the front. It was mostly on the left side, but she sometimes felt it on the right as well. It felt better in the morning and got worse throughout the day. On a scale of 1 to 10 (10 being the worst), she reported her range was 5 to 9, with the normal being around 5 in the morning and worsening to around 7 by night.

Her other health history notes were spinal stenosis in her neck; bulging discs at L3 to L5; surgeries for arthritis in her hand, a mild melanoma, and removal of an ovary. She was also experiencing pain in her legs, asthma, hay fever and allergies (dust, mold, chemical smells, etc.), indigestion (gerd), hypothyroid, high cholesterol, depression, sciatic pain, migraines, weak bladder and lactose intolerance. As you can see, there were many imbalances that her body was talking to her about.

Jessie's medications were: Levothyroxin for hypothyroid, Atorvastatin for cholesterol, Sertraline for depression, Prilosec for gerd, and Gabapentin for nerve pain. (As needed meds: Excedrin (migraines), ibuprofen (body pain), sinus meds). She saw an MD regularly for blood work to monitor the side effects of the prescription drugs.

Stress

Let me explain about a basic concept of all holistic health care practices: stress is the basis for all physical problems.

What I am talking about are the "stressors," which are the agents or conditions that cause something to be stressed. This is important so I will rephrase it: all pain, illnesses and discomforts (and again, I do mean ALL) come from our inability to handle some sort of stressor that we have been presented with, resulting in the body, mind, or spirit being overstressed. All stressors fit into one of four categories:

1) **Physical,** such as injuries, structural or genetic issues, or pathological overloads.

2) **Energetic** such as blocks or imbalances in the meridians or chakras. (Meridians carry energy through the body like arteries carry blood, and chakras carry energy into and out of the body connecting us to the world).[1, 10, 15]

3) **Emotional** such as negative or harmful belief systems (technically emotions are energetic, but they are handled differently, so I have listed them as a separate category).[5, 17, 25]

4) **Nutritional** such as not eating right, not digesting properly, or not absorbing the nutrients.[9, 27]

Finding out *what* stressor is the culprit is my job. Many times when a client has an issue for a long time (a chronic issue), we need to address all four categories in order to resolve it. This is my specialty, but I realize not many practitioners combine these different concepts into one practice. This can get very confusing and it may require working with several practitioners in order to get the skill sets needed.

The four stressors are WHAT you are correcting. HOW you correct them is simply put as:

1) **Change your habits** causing the physical stress.

2) **Strengthen energy** by balancing and unblocking it.

3) **Raise your frequency** by replacing negative emotions with positive ones.

4) **Eat right** and correct digestive issues.

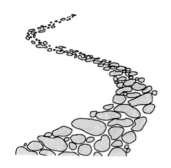

CHAPTER 2
Coming Up With a Plan

Back to Jessie's story ☞

My ultimate goal was to relieve Jessie's pain in her neck and shoulders so she could get her life back. However, with holistic care, we never know what else may need fixing in order to resolve the chief complaint. There was a lot going on and she had the pain for quite a while. Jessie does not complain easily, because I had to push her to give me information about what else was "wrong," such as the items in her health history. In holistic care, we want to know all the little details of what's going on in your body so we can pick out the right pieces of the puzzle to resolve the chief complaint.

Jessie was not familiar with energy work so that had to be introduced very slowly. As with all clients with chronic issues, I would start with the familiar and gradually lead her "getting to health" endeavor into the unfamiliarity of holistic health care. Jessie is a practicing Catholic, so I was aware I would have to fit my work into her belief systems. Jessie has a great sense of humor, which I was sure had carried her well throughout her life.

My goal for this session was to give her a massage to find her tolerance levels (✍ Perceptions) and start collecting her Body Babble signs, beginning with muscles. (✍ Body Signs)

Yep. As expected, Jessie's entire neck and shoulder top-lines, on both left and right, were so tight the muscles felt like bone. If you've ever had a muscle cramp you can imagine what this felt like. I was sure there were trigger points as well but they were buried under the hypertonic muscles. Any of the affected muscles could have caused the pain she described. (More about trigger points later in this chapter)

I did what I could with medium deep massage to relax the muscles. At the end of the session she reported less pain, more movement, and feeling "lighter." However, it did not last very long (a day), and it did seem to trigger her pain to be worse the day after. So what did the increased pain mean? The massage was too deep, but it also strongly pointed to the problem being muscular, so we had learned something. (✍ Fibro Tolerance Levels)

I also knew her shoulders, hoisted to her ears, would need some habit retraining before any lasting relief could happen. It was where she held her stress and any stress at all (pleasant or unpleasant) was likely to land right in her shoulders. It also indicated there were emotional issues involved in the forms of thought patterns, belief systems, or ingrained reactions.

*Jessie's **homework assignment** (✍ Homework) was to notice when she was raising her shoulders and give herself a few seconds to relax them. The intent was to "notice," not necessarily "fix" them at that time. Also, I asked her to investigate yoga, Tai Chi, or meditation to see if they appealed to her.*

Perceptions

I see the same types of issues over and over again. To me they are the same or similar, but the clients' perceptions are all over the map. This makes the biggest part of my job finding the right pieces of the puzzle so I can then find the way they fit together.

For example, the physical condition of a painfully tight muscle, to the practitioner, may feel the same on Client A as it does on Client B, but to the clients it feels completely different. For example, on a pain scale of 1 to 10, Client A may describe it as a level 10, where he can't function at all, and Client B may describe it as a 3 and can carry on his life fairly normally.

So to the practitioner, a pain level scale does not mean very much, but it means everything to the client. I use it for two reasons: 1) For issues that will take a while to resolve, it gives the client something to compare to that they may not have otherwise noticed because the change is so gradual. 2) It gives me a vague idea of the psychological makeup of the client as far as how they perceive pain. For example, if they tell me it's a level 3 and they can't walk, I'll approach them differently than if they tell me it's a level 9 and they are functioning normally.

Another example of perception differences is how in touch a client is with their body. One may tell me every little detail about all of her ailments (a good thing), while another may say there are no other problems. This can be because she was taught not to complain; it is easier to deal with if it stays buried; or the problem came on so gradually she is simply unaware of it. The first client type means I have to be better at managing our time together because we can easily get lost in the telling of the story. The second means I will have to be aware of the hidden issues and gently coax them into awareness and take note of any belief systems that are keeping them buried.

Body Signs

The body never lies and it is always talking to us to let us know how it is doing. You know, that person that babbles on and on about all the things that happen in their life? Just like that person, your body is talking to you all the time through pain, sensitivities, discomforts, and visible body changes. My job is to translate what it is saying by reading the acupressure points, muscle reactions, and what I call "Body Babble" signs (more on this in *Appendix A*). I palpate the acupressure points and muscle areas and label them "active" if they are uncomfortable when palpated, indicating there is stress, and "inactive" if palpating causes no discomfort, indicating all is well.

The sensitive or painful acupressure points tell me the energy is "off" in a particular meridian (meridians are vessels that carry the energy throughout the body, like arteries carry blood). Sensitivities can even indicate if it is just an energy problem or if it has gone deeper into the body to cause changes in an organ system's function.

Some muscles share nerves with the organs of the body and the muscles' reaction to palpation tells me if there is something going on with that organ system. Staying relaxed means all is well (inactive stress indicators). Tensing to protect means there is too much work to handle and the organ system is stressed (active stress indicators).[9]

By testing all the points, and adding the results to the list of Body Babble signs, I obtain a lot of puzzle pieces which I then translate into a direction for treatment. It's amazing just how talkative our bodies are, and just as amazing to me that not many people in our country know this! If you know how to listen, the incredible body will tell us when something is going wrong way in advance of any physical symptoms. It is the best preventive "medicine" there is.

More about Body Structure and Mechanics

It is very well known in the holistic realm that if your body structure is out of kilter it can cause many illnesses and pain. Muscles and bones create your structure (along with how they attach to each other, tendons and ligaments). Chiropractors and massage therapists are your go-to people to fix any structural issues. Chiropractors focus on the bone structure while massage therapists focus on the muscle structure. Bones that are out of alignment can cause muscle pain, and muscles that are asymmetrical can cause bones to be out of alignment. As you can see, they go hand in hand, so I strongly suggest you have both on your health care team. Keeping your structure in good repair can prevent a multitude of problems. If the spine is even slightly out of alignment it can cause the organ systems fed by the nerves in that area to malfunction. For example, I had muscle tension in the chest, occasional arrhythmia and pain after eating…all caused because the spine in the area between my shoulder blades was out of alignment. It was a chiropractor that rescued me.

A good massage therapist will notice (usually way ahead of any pain problems) when you are using your body in a way that could cause structural issues down the road. Spa massage therapists are usually the go-to pick if you're stressed and want help in relaxing (also excellent for moving blood, lymph, and chi). The medical, clinical, orthopedic, ART (Active Release Technique), and trigger point massage specialists are what you want for structural issues and your preventive warnings.

Trigger points are small parts of a muscle that stay contracted, forming small lumps that can refer pain to other areas that may or may not be close to where they are located. Trigger points usually form because the muscle has been overworked. For example, it is common for massage therapists to have wrist pain caused by a trigger point in the thumb. Pain in the legs is often misdiagnosed as sciatic issues when it is really caused by tightened muscle fibers in the hip.

Stretching is also a crucial part to staying structurally healthy. Here's some interesting information that many people have never thought about: it takes cell energy, called ATP, in order to relax a muscle, but none in order to contract it. Yep, that's right! It's why rigormortis sets in when we die…there is no energy there anymore so the muscles tighten. That is why, as we age, it is much harder to relax and lengthen a muscle, and that causes us to move stiffly; be less flexible; and be a bit shorter too. This means stretching is even more important than strengthening as you get closer to the golden age. I advise stretching only to the point of resistance, not to the point of pain. When it comes to lengthening a muscle, the turtle wins the race…too much too fast is asking for injury of either the muscles or the tendons.[3]

Body builders also need to stretch, because continuously strengthening a muscle will shorten it, which restricts movement and can even cause over stretching of its opposing muscle. Often I see upper back pain that is caused by the pec muscles becoming too short due to working at a computer all day. The problem is not in the back where the pain is, but in the opposing muscles in the front.

Exercise is also very important by keeping the body strong enough to easily bend, reach, balance, lift, and squat. Cardio exercise keeps the heart and vessels strong and open, helps the blood reach every tiny crevice, and moves the lymph and chi. Exercise is not my expertise, but there is so much out there you won't have any trouble finding more information.

Last, but not least, reduce your exposure to radiation. We are immersed in radiation from transmitting cell towers, phones, computers, televisions, wifi's and now watches. Do what you can to reduce their very harmful effects to your physical body. Turn off the wifi when not in use. Use the speaker on your cell phone instead of holding it up to your ear and do not carry it close to the body in pockets or bras. Do your own research to find the studies that show their damage (especially to kids and babies) so you believe it enough that you are willing to change what has become part of our everyday lives. It's about finding your own balance with it.

- -

CHALLENGE
Get an evaluation of your structure, symmetry, and muscle tone by a professional (massage therapist, chiropractor, physical thera-pist, trainer, etc.) to give you a starting point. Develop a plan and a routine to get you structurally balanced. Do not make it difficult for yourself. Lay out reasonable goals that you know are easy to reach and before you know it you'll be on the road called "steady improvement." You may want something that changes seasonally or is related to a hobby or sport to keep it interesting. The point is to make the changes one at a time so it is not overwhelming and they can become enjoyable lifestyle changes.

- -

Fibromyalgia Tolerance Levels

Everyone's tolerance to pain is different, but with fibromyalgia there is another level to this. Some clients love the deep tissue massage and it really helps them with their pain. With others, it feels great and helps for the day of the massage only to cause worse pain for the next few days after that. This makes the treatment for fibromyalgia clients particularly difficult to find the balance of "just enough." With any client who is more sensitive, there are techniques that can be used to enhance bodywork without having to go too deep for their comfort (such as heat, energy work, or do less more often).

Homework

This "getting there" process is not something I "do" to you—this process is self-empowering, so there is a lot of homework as part of the retraining process of muscle memory, beliefs, reactions, and eating habits. I attempt to space out the homework so it is not over-whelming, and by the time I am adding more, the old assignments have become habits and don't require as much thought.

It does not matter whom you are seeing about your health, everyone should give you information about how you can help yourself. If they don't tell you, ASK! And while we're at it, PLEASE take charge of your own health. Do your own research, consult with those in-the-know, and make your own informed decisions that you have confidence in. Our medical world is so specialized, there often is no one practitioner taking all the different aspects of a problem into account, thus, leaving that up to you. So, I am assigning all of you homework right now—learn about holistic care and what fits well with you.

Now! Before you need it. Because it is preventative.

Now! Because if you do get sick, you will be too tired and too scared to learn it…then you'll get trapped on our medical system's train of pharmaceuticals.

Back to Jessie's story ☞

We had checked out Jessie's physical issues, and next was to see if Jessie was getting enough nutrients so her body could heal—without fuel, the work cannot be done. I did this through palpating certain muscles and acupressure points. Let's just say Jessie had more points active than not, so she was clearly not getting the nutrients her body needed. Her diet was fair to good, but her system was either not breaking the food down, not absorbing enough nutrients, or both. Also, one of her physical symptoms, mild water retention, indicated proteins may be an issue, which was an additional sign of long-term stress for the digestive system. This was a process to work through and correct, and at the time, I only did the preliminary check to see if we needed to go further. The answer was a resounding, "Yes."

There were also signs of unresolved emotional issues that were keeping the stress levels high for many years (chronic stress).

Jessie's Body Signs of Chronic Stress

- *Raised shoulders*
- *Chest breathing*
- *Stilted speech at times (an unusual number and oddly placed pauses)*
- *Weakened energy in spleen, pancreas, liver, kidneys, and adrenals*
- *Fatigue and depression*

Jessie's additional **homework** *was to lightly stretch her neck in all six directions one to two times per day—note I said lightly! That meant to only go to the point of resistance (NOT to the point of pain or discomfort) and to hold for only five seconds.*

Also, to get her digestion corrections started, I suggested the following:

- *Take full spectrum digestive enzymes with each meal to help break down the food for more complete digestion and to*

help take some of the load off her pancreas. "Full spectrum"
will include amylase, protease, lipase, and cellulase. Jessie par-
ticularly needs protease to help her breakdown of protein.

- *Eat more fresh, organic fruits and vegetables.*
- *Cut back on the sugar (it turns out Jessie had a sweet tooth).*
- *Breathe with the belly instead of the chest. (✍ Chest Breathing)*

Conclusion

Jessie had many things going on and was clearly not getting the nutrients
she needed to support the stress she carried. Until the stress and the
nutrition were addressed, the pain would most likely keep returning.
The findings that supported this were:

- *reported relief after massage that did not continue for long;*
- *improved muscle condition without reported pain improve-*
  ment;
- *prolonged stress symptoms;*
- *active stress indicators for digestion;*
- *active stress indicators through the acupressure points.*

We went over the plan, the budget, and the time available. Jessie
was enthusiastic and hopeful about finally having a solution to her
pain. As she left she reported her pain level around 4 which told me
she was reacting to the energy of the plan and therefore gave me an
even higher confidence level that we were on the right track.

We set up appointments for every other week instead of every
week because Jessie was very diligent about doing her homework and
it would be easier on her wallet and her schedule. Our plan was to
continue addressing all stressors: physical muscle issues and posture
changes, energetic imbalances (including emotional), and incomplete
digestion and diet. We would take each session as it came and rely on

her body signs and symptoms to decide which category took precedence at that time. (✍ Making a Plan)

Chest Breathing

Breathing is the most important nourishment we give to our bodies. We can get along without water for a few days, without food for a few weeks, but without air we start to die after a few minutes. In spite of this fact, few of us think much about our breathing. So please do your body a favor and read on....

Breathing brings in oxygen and expels carbon dioxide—we all learned this in biology class—but, it also expels other toxins, moves and invigorates energy, cools and warms, and has an effect on our skin, immune system, digestion, strength, meridians, and chakras.

Our bodies are built to handle stress, but they are not built to handle the sustained stress that today's society imposes on us. Stress without sufficient relaxation and play leads to muscle "habits" that do not go away and we are often unaware of them. One of these habits is "chest breathing."

Normal breathing uses the diaphragm to move the abdomen out with an in-breath and in with an out-breath (this can feel like it is your abdominal muscles doing the work). Watch any animal or baby sleeping and you'll see the belly move, but not the ribs. If your shoulders move up and/or your ribs get wider when breathing in, you are chest breathing. This is perfectly normal when you are under stress of any kind (physical, mental, or emotional), because chest breathing is your turbo charge for air. If you chest breathe all the time, you have no turbo charge when you need it. The lower parts of the lungs have even been known to atrophy (waste away) because of many years of non-use due to chest breathing.

So breathe normally (with your belly) and use the ribs and chest to add extra when you need it. This has many benefits:

- It keeps the stomach energy moving down which prevents heartburn, indigestion, hiatal hernias, and sometimes headaches. It also may correct these problems if they already exist.
- It helps to prevent weakness in the arms and legs because the lungs are a major energy "pump" that keeps the energy moving throughout the body.
- It can help with high blood pressure, headaches, or muscle pain in the upper back, shoulders or neck because chest breathing forces the energy to stay in your upper body. This can also cause a tight feeling that can feel like a mild heart attack and lead to heart palpitations.
- It brings energy down to your center in your belly where it can be directed (with your thoughts and intent) to energize and heal.
  - Breathe in, using your full lung capacity and imagine it a storehouse of energy, then breathe out and visualize that energy going to wherever you need it.
  - For aerobics, visualize sparkles of energy filling your lungs, then spreading throughout your body, nourishing, feeding and energizing it.
  - For illnesses, picture the breath nourishing the organ systems affected.
  - For extra strength visualize the energy moving through your muscles as you breathe in for contraction and out for release.

If you are currently chest breathing, practice and practice until you catch yourself breathing abdominally without having to think about it. And, when you are under stress, remind yourself to breathe deep into the belly to prevent the chest breathing from becoming a habit.

Making a Plan

I found it is fruitless to make detailed plans because it is better to let the body lead…it has been right more often than any attempt at detailed plans I made. Knowing what needs to be addressed is enough to get started. It is best to let what presents itself to be the guide to which of the issues are to be worked on during a particular session. Obviously, if there is no practitioner that can work with all four stressors (physical, energetic, emotional, nutritional), the client will have to determine the order-of-go, and making a plan becomes more necessary. This is where it is imperative that the practitioners be willing to work together to help their client in this process.

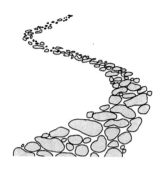

CHAPTER 3
Getting Started

Back to Jessie's story ☞

In the third visit, I noticed Jessie's shoulders were more relaxed during our pre-session discussion, but they instantly tensed when there was anything, even slightly agitating, to talk about. In keeping with my previous decision to lighten the massage so it would not elicit the pain, I used hot stones and energy to warm the muscles so I could accomplish the same with less pressure. This time there were fewer trigger points, and her neck movement was considerably improved. Jessie reported there was significant pain relief after this session that lasted until she did some heavy lifting during household chores that same evening.

I took note that previous to this session, Jessie reported her overall pain level was around 5 in the morning and 7 by evening. In spite of improved muscle tonicity, she was experiencing no pain relief as yet.

I introduced the energy work (by using reiki and acupressure) to ground her and to correct the energy flow through her shoulders. The muscles were then responding better to the lighter massage and trigger point work.

It was time to start the shift in belief systems, and for this, I needed to know what tools she already had and used. While I was doing the muscle work I asked Jessie more about her religious beliefs. (✍ Religions) She receives comfort from prayer and the teachings of The Bible, and believes she has guides (or guardian angels) and deceased relatives and friends visiting to help.

I also needed to know the depth of Jessie's religious beliefs that would give me a good indication of her feelings of self-worth. So sticking with her religion, I asked if she felt she had "the right" to call in her spiritual "heavy hitters" for help, such as archangels, ascended masters, Jesus, saints, or God Himself. (✍ Strengthening Intent) Fortunately, she already felt worthy of such help and comfortable asking for it, so this made the job much easier, because unworthiness can be a very deep issue and trust in her faith could help strengthen her intentions of getting well. She had a great toolbox already that she could use to start her journey of "belief system correction."

I was quite surprised when another quandary came up in this session. For some reason Jessie's MD instructed her to NOT take the enzymes.

"Why?"

"She doesn't believe in them."

"Did she happen to mention why?"

I never did find out. (✍ Digestion and Enzymes)

However, Jessie decided on her own to take them anyway. I would have discussed this with her doctor, but Jessie was okay with us being on different pages for this particular decision. (✍ Why Holistic Health Care is so Hard)

While working through this session, I noticed Jessie seemed calmer if I repeated the grounding acupressure points. So for **homework,** *I gave her instructions to ground at least one time per day. (✍ Grounding)*

I suggested removing gluten from her diet as a test to see if it would make a difference. (✍ Wheat, Sugar and GMOs) I did not press it at that time because she was already working on reducing sugar, but I put it out there to at least plant the seed.

Additional homework was to notice when she was in rest-restore mode (PSNS) and when she was in fight-flight mode (SNS), and take note of her emotions at that time. (✑ The Nervous System—SNS and PSNS)

We also went over how she was doing on her past homework assignments.

Progress of Homework Assignments

For Energy and Emotions:

- *Notice when she is raising her shoulders—she noticed she is doing it a lot.*
- *Investigate yoga, Tai Chi, or meditation—she is going to try a yoga DVD she already has.*
- *NEW: ground every day.*

For Physical:

- *Stretch her neck—she reported this is not going well because she didn't think she was doing it right, so didn't do it for fear of making it worse. We reviewed the instructions, and I had her do it herself a few times until she was comfortable.*
- *NEW: notice when she is in rest/relax mode and when in fight/flight mode.*

For Digestion:

- *Digestive enzymes—she is doing ok with this, but just starting to remember to take them consistently.*
- *Eat more fruits and vegetables, less sugar—she said, "I'm trying!"*
- *NEW: think about removing gluten and pay attention to how her body responds to the thought. Does she retract from it or move towards it?*

Religions

I deal with belief systems…a lot! And, there are none more deeply held than religious beliefs…they can form our life, and therefore, our health. Many beliefs help us to be better people, while others can cause life long problems. Religions have done much to help people better themselves, but they have also done a lot of harm. Helping people discern which is which can be a tricky business because the beliefs are held so dear.

It is time to change the low frequency beliefs that religions have taught and that have evolved through the ages to influence our deep core belief systems.

When we realize that something we have thought to be true for a long time turns out not to be, it is natural to search for blame. However, that serves no one, especially ourselves. I believe this list below to be of low frequency beliefs based on who we are as a people today. Ages ago, when these ideas were introduced, they probably were needed to raise the frequency of the people of that time. We have evolved and it is simply time for us to set a higher bar.

- We are born in sin.
- If you do not repent you will go to hell.
- You are not worthy enough to communicate directly with God.
- People will be tested by God and tempted by the devil.
- You are not smart enough to make your own choices so you must do as your religious leaders tell you.
- Going against the beliefs of the religion means you are condemned.
- It's okay to judge as wrong those who have different religious beliefs.
- You should feel guilty. (This one can be very subtle. I consider it the sneakiest and most obtrusive controlling mechanism of all.)

These are beliefs that are very energetically damaging to our health and it's my job to help people find their power, get rid of their guilt, learn when they are judging, and feel equal to all others at the same time respecting their religious beliefs (so the baby doesn't get tossed out with the bath water). As a non-denominational parson, I don't always get it right, but I find the balance as best I can.

- -

CHALLENGE

Can you add some of your own low frequency beliefs to the above examples? You may have winced a bit as your read them, but imagine how your thinking would change if you did NOT believe any of them. Would your attitude (and life) improve? If others shed these beliefs would your life improve?

Do NOT look yet, but next I have listed what high frequency beliefs could replace the above list. BEFORE PEEKING I'd like you to think about it for a bit; add to and subtract from the list above to make it your own; and come up with your own affirmations that fit you. However, if you would like some ideas, you may peek at the list coming up next.

- -

Changing Religious Beliefs

- We are born in sin.
  - We are born with lessons to learn in this life.
- If you do not repent, you will go to hell.
  - My mistakes teach me—I learn from them and move on as a better person.
- You are not worthy enough to speak directly to God.
  - I am no more or no less worthy than any other person, including clergy and authority figures.

- People will be tested by God and tempted by the devil.
  - We live in a dual reality with opposing sides that balance each other (yin and yang). I create "me" with the choices I make with what is presented to me...every minute of every day.
- You are not smart enough to make your own choices so you must do as your religious leaders tell you.
  - I choose which suggestions given to me that I will follow. My discernment in these choices creates "me."
- Going against the beliefs of the religions means you are condemned.
  - We all have free will. The religion I have chosen is the one that helps me improve "me" the best, but I choose, always, what is right and wrong for me.
- It's okay to judge as wrong those who have different religious beliefs.
  - I respect different opinions about how to become a better person, and I respect the rights of others to believe in different religions that help them do that.
- You should feel guilty. (This is the sneakiest and most obtrusive controlling mechanism of all).
  - I recognize guilt as a message to look at what I have done and make changes. Guilt has no use after that so I let it go.

Strengthening Intent [2, 12, 22]

The intent you send out to the universe adds strength to the probability of that intent becoming reality. So strengthening your intent is important and both quantity and quality can help it along. Your intent needs to be clearly stated and felt:

- Write it down because the written word has power too.[16]

- Make sure it is about what you want and not what you don't want.[22]
- Think about your intent and get into the feeling of it as if it has already come true.
- Repeat this daily

The stronger we set our intent and the clearer we are about it, the more energy the universe has to create the people, events, and spaces to bring it into manifestation. This is what vision boards, affirmations and positive thinking are all about.

I find that the action of asking for help assists in focusing the mind to the intent because it compels you to define it better and, while you are doing that, you usually have a much more concentrated focus as well.

This can be as simple as explaining it to a friend and asking them to imagine it happening for you. The help can come from objects with like properties, such as crystals and essential oils.[7, 11] It can come from symbols or icons. Or, if you believe in help from the other side, it can come from animal totems, guides, and entities who represent the energy of your intent. Asking for help from your religion's supernatural beings can bring an emotional component to the intent, which strengthens the energy of it even further.

Symbols and icons are examples of talismans that gain energetic strength just because of the number of people that think the same way about them. Another way to put this: thoughts become "thought forms" which become part of the cosmic energy. Every time someone has the same thought it adds to the strength of that thought form, and eventually it becomes mass consciousness and a definitive part of our reality. Examples of this are the cross, the menorah, or even a stop sign. If enough people believe they have power or deep meaning, then they do because the sight of them invokes an emotion and even if it is a very subtle emotion, it is sent out into the universe and adds strength to that collective consciousness. Talismans can generate positive (high frequency) feelings, or negative (low frequency) feelings. Just think of the emotions the swastika invokes in people and you will know what I mean.

You can create your own talismans for each new thing you want to manifest. Any object will work, but stone, crystal, and bone are great at storing energy. Spend some meditation time with the object, thinking about what you are creating, imagining what it is like…feel it, know it, smell it, taste it, hear it, and see it, as if you already have it. Command (as in "co-manifest") that this intent be cast to the universe and to the object. Do this three separate times, then put the object in a place where you will see it often. Even when you don't notice it anymore, your subconscious will pick up the vibrations of your intent every time you pass by it, think about it, or carry it in your pocket. (✍ Conscious vs Subconscious)

An example of the importance of intent was given to me by my horse, Squire. He was used to acupressure and very communicative about what he felt he needed and what he didn't. I was attempting to work the Spleen-21 point and he kept moving away from me…an indication he didn't want it. I intuitively knew (or so I thought) he needed it, so tried other means such as switching hands or giving him space and trying again. He didn't want any of it. I then remembered I had set my intent to help balance the spleen meridian, but this point is also very good at unblocking energy anywhere in the body. I restated my intent to be about unblocking, and Squire leaned into me, clearly wanting the work on that point.

So always, always, make your intent clear to the universe no matter what you are doing, whether it's baking a cake or changing your life.

Digestion and Enzymes [9]

Any pain, illness, discomfort, or emotional issue may have its root cause in insufficient nutrients to the cells, which diminishes them from functioning properly. There have even been highly publicized research articles about the relationship between gut health and a number of emotional and brain issues, including depression, anxiety, and autism.

Our cells need food to work, just like our car needs gas to run. The process of food intake, breakdown, absorption, and elimination is called digestion and it's what delivers the nutrients to the cells so they can function and thrive, creating a vibrant you. As much as we would like to ignore the physical requirements of our bodies and eat and do anything we want, we all know we will not last as long if we do (i.e. be dead sooner).

The system can malfunction at any one of these four stages of process. It is my job to help you determine if it is malfunctioning, and if so, what is not getting the right nutrients to thrive, and which process is failing and why. Then I put together a plan for correcting it.

Digestion or nutritional problems most often cause tender areas in the muscles that share the same nerves as the digestive organs. When the body is balanced and digestion problems healed, the pain, ticklishness, or tender areas go away. Palpating these areas and tracking the changes lets us know whether we are on the right path towards radiant health…or not, then we know to change course.

There is an old saying, "Good digestion then good recovery," meaning your chances of recovery are far better after surgery, illnesses or injury if your body can get the nutrients to the cells. In Chinese medicine, with any major problem, the stomach energy is checked first to get an understanding of the body's constitutional ability to heal.

Many times, when the digestion system is not running up to par, we face a bigger problem because it's a catch 22 cycle that is more difficult to get turned around—you need the nutrients to heal the digestive system, but you can't get the nutrients until the digestive system is healed. This is the trap we encounter whenever our allopathic medical system overlooks the cause by only treating the symptoms

The only way, other than energetic work (that I have found anyway), to heal a failing digestive system is to get the nutrients into your body by "bypassing" it. The only way I know of to do this, short of intravenous feeding, is to use enzymes. Enzymes are those itty-bitty things that break things down. They have two functions: digestive and metabolic.

Digestive enzymes are found both in food (food enzymes) and in our body's digestive system (digestive enzymes). The food enzymes are already in the food we eat (or should be) and they help break it down so it will rot and return to dirt (which is why strawberries didn't last very long). However, this is a problem if you want to ship food across the country, so most of it no longer contains any food enzymes. They've been removed to lengthen their shelf life (which is why strawberries dry out instead of rot). Also, heating and radiation destroys food enzymes. (Note: Cooking (heat) and microwaving (radiation) affect enzymes, but do not necessarily affect the vitamins and minerals.)

Now, for the real problem: our pancreas has to make up for these missing food enzymes by producing more digestive enzymes every time we eat and this is extra work it was not born to do for an entire lifetime. Sometimes? Of course. It can handle sometimes, but not as often as our Standard American Diet requires.

Metabolic enzymes are the instigators for the many chemical processes our bodies need to function (chemical processes such as producing and repairing cells, creating energy, and clearing toxins). Metabolic enzymes are found throughout the entire body, and many bodily functions depend on enzymes.

What helps with extracting minerals out of our food? Enzymes. What starts the process of making hydrochloric acid? Enzymes. What sparks cells into action? Enzymes. What helps clear the debris? Enzymes. What instigates energy to be made from fat? Enzymes. What helps insulin do its job? Enzymes. This list of what they do is very long and the pancreas produces many of them (as well as the hormones insulin and glucagon which help regulate blood sugar). If we keep the pancreas busy by eating all the time and eating foods that have no food enzymes, the pancreas may not keep up with its job of producing metabolic enzymes and hormones, because it's too busy producing digestive enzymes. What could go wrong then? Anything! This is why good digestion is so important. Just think about the increase in diabetes and how the overworked pancreas contributes to it. Good digestion then good recovery.

Wheat, Sugar, and GMOs

In my opinion, we should all stay far away from wheat, sugar, and all genetically modified organisms (GMOs). The grain, wheat, is in a very large portion of our foods…breads, cereals, pastries, etc., and is used as a filler or thickener in just about everything.

Wheat used to be processed more slowly without chemicals, which allowed it to produce its own enzymes that helped the body break it down and release the nutrients. Today's processing does not allow this enzyme production, and making matters worse, it allows the spraying of toxic weed-killers. This combination makes it very difficult for our bodies to recognize what wheat is and digest it (and consequently few nutrients are utilized from it). It then can become a form of poison to the body (especially for people with leaky gut), creating fatigue, achiness, pain, depression, a weak immune system, or worse, auto-immune diseases.

Gluten is the gluey stuff in wheat, rye, barley, and spelt that makes it stick together when wet, and it's the part that becomes the most poisonous. Anyone with gluten intolerance, or celiac disease needs to stay away from any type of gluten because even the tiniest amount can raise havoc for months. This I know from experience.

I had been subjected to bronchitis for five years, and the doctors could find no reason for it. They said things like, "You're getting older you know," and, "That's what you get for living in upstate New York." The last time I had it, I was coughing up a considerable amount of blood and had become so weak I could not hold my arms over my head long enough to do my hair. I was gray and pale, had no ambition, and felt nauseous most of the time. I knew if I didn't find the answer, it would kill me. I started looking beyond our medical system and found a kinesiologist who told me that wheat gluten was the cause.

"WHAT!?"

"Bread?"

"The staple of life?"

This was in 1995, before the general public knew much about it. Having nothing to lose, I cut gluten from my diet and began feeling better within a couple of weeks. I excitedly went back to my doctor to tell him I found the problem! He did not want to know. That was the final straw that forced me to give up on our allopathic medical system and continue finding out-of-the-box answers. It took me a couple of years to get gluten completely out of my life because it seemed like it was in everything. I slowly learned to check things like toothpaste, hair spray, lotions and cosmetics. Fortunately, availability of gluten free products has greatly improved since then.

I am grateful for this experience and the unwillingness of my doctor to acknowledge it because it turned out to be the start of my new radiantly healthy body and subsequently my new career.

Sugar is another big culprit in ill health, especially artificial sweeteners. Our bodies have no idea what to do with artificial sweeteners, so they are sent to the liver to be broken down for elimination. People who drink a can or two of diet soda a day can end up with a liver that looks just like an advanced alcoholic's…full of sclerosis.[23]

I have known many people who had annoying joint pain that went away completely when they stopped consuming artificial sweeteners. Also, in the past few years, studies have shown they have the undesirable effect of weight gain. So, if you want a soda, have one with real sugar, but keep the overall sugar intake down to less than 40 grams per day.

I had been a sugar junkie since I could remember. I could not get enough of the stuff, especially if it was in the form of chocolate. I've learned that for me sugar is fine, but only in moderation. Through my efforts to find my balance with it, my intake quantity was up and down enough that I was able to get a very clear picture of all areas in my body and life that are affected by it. It's an impressive list!

My Areas Affected by Too Much Sugar

Eyesight	Allergies	Ambition
Breathing	Edema	Enthusiasm
Teeth / Gums	Blood Pressure	Choices
Immune System	Weight	Happiness
Sleep		Grocery Budget

GMOs are genetically modified organisms and there are very conflicting research studies about whether they are safe for us or not. Most of the grains grown in the USA now are GMOs. Many countries have banned them. Humans have grown up with grains for thousands of years...we've had GMOs for only a few in comparison. As for me, I avoid them because they are not grains to the human body—they are "unknowns," and the body rejects "unknowns" as invaders. The studies I've read are inconclusive about what this will do to our long-term health. So, find your own balance of consumption with it that you feel comfortable with.

How the Stomach Works

The stomach is small, shrunken, and empty in its relaxed state. When we eat something, it enters the stomach causing it to stretch to accommodate the amount of food. The stomach is located just below the sternum (breast bone) and this part of the abdomen will expand, causing our pants to feel tighter. The food stays here for 45–60 minutes while it churns the food into smaller pieces and continues the digestion of carbohydrates (starches, grains, and sugars) with the enzyme called amylase that was produced in the mouth and swallowed with the food.

The stomach begins the process of creating HCL (hydrochloric acid, or stomach acid) which is then used to create pepsin, a type of protease which breaks down proteins into usable form (amino acids). This is the process interrupted by antacid medications. In the meantime, it has communicated to the pancreas to get busy making the other digestive enzymes needed. This process takes about 45 minutes, so the stomach has all that time to break down the food into smaller pieces and to continue digestion of carbohydrates with the enzymes that came with the food itself and with the enzymes from the glands in the mouth. However, once the HCL is made, the stomach contents become very acidic, carbohydrate breakdown no longer happens, and the protein breakdown begins.

What does all this mean? There are four points to take away from this information:

1) If you graze throughout the day (continuous snacking and drinking), it causes the stomach to be working all the time and the acid to be present in the stomach all the time. This inhibits the digestion of carbohydrates as well as stresses the pancreas (which can result in reduced enzyme production for other vital functions of the body). For this reason, **give your stomach and pancreas enough rest**...allow at least three hours between eating or drinking (anything except water).

2) **Don't snack** while you are making your meal, because that starts the 45 minute countdown. Coffee, teas, fruit juices and such are all treated as food...only water passes through to the intestines without starting the process.

3) **Chew your food thoroughly** so more amylase is produced in the mouth and the stomach has less "churning" to do to make the food into smaller pieces.

4) **Drink room temperature water** with your meals, not ice water. Enzymes need a certain temperature range in order to work. Therefore, very cold or very hot foods change the temperature of the stomach enough that it stops the digestion function of enzymes. This causes undigested foods to be passed on to the intestines, which can cause many toxic conditions.

Our digestive system is designed to eat foods that contain their own enzymes and to make those that are missing in the food.

Our current SAD (Standard American Diet) contains very few enzymes, if any. Heating and radiating food kills them, as well as many pesticides, herbicides, and processing methods that inhibit or destroy their ability to function. Even most of our organic and raw foods have been radiated. The only solution to this is to take enzyme supplements to replace those that are no longer there naturally. If you are choosing a supplement, make sure it contains all three major categories of food breakdown, amylase (carbohydrates), protease (proteins), and lipase (fats) as well as cellulase for assisting with raw vegetables.

You do not need to be a fanatic about any of these suggestions, but, if you have digestion issues, try them out to see if they help.

More About Nutrition [9]

The list below describes the basics for nutrition. Forget the fad diets and move slowly towards these ideas. Unless you are in crisis, there is no need to do this in a hurry...I've found more permanent results come when new habits have time to slowly sink in.

1) Eat the right foods. That means lots of vegetables and fruits and much less meat, carbohydrates, sugars, and caffeine than the Standard American Diet. Modern food processing destroys many nutrients. Even when eating the "right" foods we are taking in less nutrients than past times. On top of that, we are ingesting the toxins they are grown with such as pesticides, herbicides, and coatings for bugs and appearance. (Egads! It's so easy to lull ourselves into a false sense of security.) **Organic and raw** is best (if you can digest them). If you believe you are eating well and still have physical or emotional issues, then seek out someone who can help you determine what is lacking or in excess.

Your body will tell you—all you need is to listen to the signs and translate the message.

2) You may be eating it, but your body may not be getting it, and that is just like not eating it at all. The Standard American Diet (SAD—and it is sad) does not contain the enzymes required to break the food down so we can actually digest it and absorb it. Cooking, radiation and other atrocities like pesticides and herbicides destroy enzymes (as well as some of the vitamins and minerals). So, **getting the enzymes is important!** (You have already read about them in the Digestion and Enzymes section, so I won't go into it again here.)[9]

3) The other thing that's destroyed with cooking and chemicals is the probiotics. Probiotics are the friendly bacteria that live in the gut, which, by the way, can be severely compromised when you take antibiotics. Probiotics help maintain the gut lining which prevents contaminants from entering the body. They also destroy many of the unwanted toxins passing through the gut. These functions not only assist with digestion, but also assist the endocrine system, the nervous system, and the immune system (especially when it comes to the inflammatory response). This is believed to be due to the many detectors in the gut that are the interface between our environment and other parts of the body.

So again, in today's world, most of us need to make sure **probiotics** are part of our nutrition intake when needed. The best form is raw and organic foods that have not been radiated, and fermented foods. If you're having lots of intestinal issues, it can take anywhere from 1 to 6 months to fully replenish the probiotics in the gut. Once this is done, most people do not need to continue taking them because they will reproduce in the gut on their own (providing you don't take any anti-biotics).

4) Another big problem with the SAD, is the imbalance of the essential fatty acids that are required to make hormones, and to absorb some of the vitamins (among other things). Hormones regulate ALL bodily functions, so it's vital to our health to make sure we have the right fat in our diet. With the SAD, we generally get plenty of omega-6, but we do not get enough **omega-3 fat** to balance it, thus putting our health at risk. So, think "fat is good"…it just has to be the right kind of fat, such as, coconut oil, extra virgin olive oil, flax seeds, grape seed oil, or hemp seeds to name a few.[8]

5) **Antioxidants** are part of your cleanup crew and they make sure the "wrong" things don't grow too fast, and the "right" things break down slowly. (More about "cleanup crew" in Chapter 4.) The word "oxidants" can be confusing because cells need oxygen to live, and it sounds like "antioxidants" means "anti-oxygen," which is not the case. Oxidizing is a process of breaking down the cells with what is called "free-radicals" (left over oxygen electrons). Cancer is an example of what too many free radicals can cause. This means we need lots of antioxidant rich foods (like blue berries, beans, artichokes, russet potatoes, and wolfberries) in our diets to help with the cleaning up life's debris.

6) **Eliminate the chemicals**…especially artificial sweeteners because they can only be metabolized by your liver, which puts a huge strain on your whole system. Plus studies have shown that they encourage your body to gain weight… the opposite of what you are probably using them for. GMOs (genetically modified foods) are not recognized by the body either. Studies have shown that animals fed

only GMO food die. There are no studies that I could find that show they are safe over long periods of time. And, as written above, it is best to eat organically grown food to eliminate pesticides and herbicides, which are known poisons.

7) **Maintain an alkaline PH level.** Diseases and cancer love an acidic environment to live in while body cells love an alkaline environment. If your body is alkaline, viruses, bacteria, funguses, and cancer have a hard time surviving. It's easy to check—urinate in a cup first thing in the morning before eating and dip a PH test strip in it (available in most drug stores). If it registers around 6.7 or above, in the green/blue range, you are fine (alkaline). If you are below that in the yellow to orange color you may be too acidic, so start paying attention. A proper diet, as mentioned above (especially more leafy greens, and cutting back on meats, dairy, caffeine, and sugars) should maintain an alkaline level. There are many products on the market to help you switch from acid to alkaline. You can also put baking soda in water (about one teaspoon) before going to bed to give yourself a boost. I consider this a band-aid to get you through a rough spot because I found no studies about long-term use.

8) **Drink enough water.** Water is second to air in how long we can live without it. Air is measured in minutes, water in days, and food in weeks. Water is constantly being depleted through breath, sweat, and evaporation, so the need to replenish it is continuous. Water conducts electricity which helps our cells communicate with each other and our chi flow. It allows the blood and lymph to run through

the vessels and carry nutrients and waste. It also contains hydrogen and oxygen which are used in chemical processes within the body. Without it, the body is a pile of dust. If you get moderate exercise the recommended amount per day is $^1/_2$ your weight in ounces. If you get little exercise, I've found $^1/_3$ will do. Increasing water intake for those deficient is the first thing I recommend for eliminating muscle and joint pain.

9) Pay attention to the additional suggestions made in the "How the Stomach Works" section above.

That's it! If you can follow these basic rules, you are way ahead of the game concerning your health. It's not so hard.

- -

CHALLENGE

Using the nine suggestions, lay out a step-by-step plan for "getting there" within a year. Start with whichever one is easiest for you, then add another one in six to seven weeks. That will give you plenty of time to change your habits and make it part of your new healthier life.

- -

Why Holistic Health Care is so Hard

The conflicting advice between Jessie's doctor and me about enzymes is a typical example of what clients run into when working with holistic practitioners. And, it's SO CONFUSING to everyone! This is why it's important for the client to be their own advocate and understand that each practitioner is coming from their training and their life experiences and in many cases both can be right about the same subject at the same time, even when it seems like opposing views.

Doctors (to date anyway) have been trained in their fields of pharmaceuticals, surgery, and treating symptoms. The idea that you can fix a problem with food, thoughts, and bodywork is foreign to many of them. Numerous doctors have even been taught that holistic care is to be avoided, and this is reinforced by insurance companies' lack of payment for it. Add to that the doctors' concern of lawsuits and that their liability insurance will not cover them if they don't do "what all the other doctors are doing," and you have huge resistance to change to new or different ideas.

It is my opinion we are in the biggest and most rapid transition the world has ever seen. There are those in the old paradigm camp, those in the new, and those making their way from old to new (from physical as the basis of existence to energy as the basis of existence). This has been creating conflict and chaos for a long time. It started in the sixties (remember the flower children?); reached its height in 2012 (when the chaos really began); and will start to smooth out through the twenties and thirties (again, my opinion based on much reading). The entire world has to change from one way of thinking (to put it simply, fear and war) to the complete opposite way of thinking (cooperation and love). This is a massive undertaking, so be patient with those out there you don't agree with, especially when it comes to your own health. Be open, listen to the differing opinions, then listen to your gut…it will not lie to you.

If you are following holistic care, respect the decision of those who are not because change is not for everyone. Also, if you wish to continue down the allopathic path, respect those who choose energy medicine because it is valid, real and based in science.

Grounding

Grounding is so important, especially in today's chaotic world. We are in physical bodies and they need to stay connected to the physical earth in order to stay in equilibrium. Otherwise, you may feel like your thoughts are chaotic, feel a bit spacey, continuously be in manic mode, or not be able to stay in the easy flow of life.

There are many ways to stay grounded, such as sitting on the ground (gardening is great!), biomats, meditation, essential oils[11], yoga, crystals[7], and others.

- -

CHALLENGE

This is the meditation I gave Jessie…go ahead and try it:

- Sit or stand quietly.
- Focus on relaxing.
- Visualize a beautiful braided cord (any colors that resonate with you) and add a crystal at the end.
- Picture this cord coming out your feet, going all the way to the center of the earth and the crystal going firmly into place (kurchunk!).
- Then thank the earth for accepting you.
- Repeat this to ground your heart to the sun—imagine a beautiful cord from your heart connecting you to the sun.
- Once you do it a few times, it only takes a few seconds, so do it often.

It's important not to force it, because everyone is different. If you can't visualize it, just pay attention to what has popped into your mind and follow it. What's it telling you? Did you see a different type of cord? Different colors? Did it not want to go all the way to the center? As an example, with one of my clients, as I attempted to visualize the cord dropping to the center of the earth, I saw it flinging out to my left. Huh? So, I let that happen, relaxed my mind, and followed the cord. It went to the Rocky Mountains! For her, grounding to the mountains was better. For another client, the cord was rejected by the earth and flung back at her. Again, huh? For her there was a belief that the devil lived there and her subconscious wanted no part of connecting to it. Just this acknowledgment released that thought form and she then grounded easily.

- -

The Nervous System—SNS and PSNS

Our subconscious is what runs our lives, and it does so with learned behavior. The conscious mind can think, reason, and make decisions, but it runs a very tiny portion of our everyday life.

Our world, our perceptions, our lives are created based on the energy frequencies our subconscious minds are continuously emitting and reacting to, even in sleep state.

The sympathetic nervous system (SNS) is in charge of our "flight or fight" responses, and the parasympathetic nervous system (PSNS) is in charge of our "rest and restore" responses. These two systems balance back and forth, keeping us in equilibrium. When SNS is sustained for long periods (sustained stress), we become very sensitive to the stimulus that invokes it—sometimes to the point of "any little thing" will trigger an SNS response. This is sometimes referred to as post-traumatic stress syndrome (PTSD), and, it's not just being in a war that can create this. It can be a stressful job, a stressful relationship, or simply a belief system that tells our body it is not safe.

Eventually our body will say, "I can't sustain this anymore!" and PSNS will take over creating extreme rest and restoration, which our society interprets as depression.

Normally SNS and PSNS keep us in equilibrium by moving from one to the other in a gentle teeter-totter fashion. When sustained stress causes us to stay in SNS for long periods, the gentle teeter-totter can become a wild roller coaster ride swinging from full hyper-speed to deep depression. Allopathic medicine interprets this as bi-polar.

Knowledge of these concepts is the basis for changing our lives and changing it faster than you may think possible. Is it instantaneous? Sometimes, but usually not. It's usually an educational journey that is both joyful and hard at times. However, it will be filled with hope, and it just may give you back control of your life and how you create it.

What does it take? Simply put, a willingness to change, and a willingness to do the work to make it happen. There are five categories of tasks that will give you an idea of what it will take:

1) **Rethinking:** Sometimes it's a simple belief system adjustment such as, "It's hard to find a job," to "It's easy to find a job."

2) **Retraining:** Sometimes it's a retraining of the subconscious from "I react this way to said stimulus," to "Now I react this other way."

3) **Releasing:** Sometimes it's uncovering the subtle emotion that is hidden from awareness, so it can resolve and exit the body cells leaving them to function more normally. There are many methods besides mine that can accomplish this, such as Meridian Tapping (EFT) and Heart Based Therapy (HBT).

4) **Balancing:** Sometimes it's convincing your nervous system to calm and balance—"It is safe, so relax." This can be accomplished by stimulating the PSNS through energy work while you are thinking of a situation that normally invokes an SNS reaction—"Not safe...RUN." I use a combination of massage, acupressure, essential

oils, heart work, and intuition to facilitate this. Often the methods for Releasing also work for Balancing.

5) **Unblocking:** Sometimes it's unblocking stagnant energy so it can properly nourish the body system in charge of the reaction. Blocked energy can be caused by inactivity, cut meridians, or scar tissue; and effective ways to correct it are massage, acupressure, acupuncture, yoga, and martial arts.

...and sometimes it's all of the above.

Conscious and Subconscious

It is important that our conscious and subconscious stay in synch with each other. These are the facts:

- We are creative beings and we create our lives and realities whether we are aware of it or not.
- It is our subconscious minds that create our everyday lives.
- The subconscious is learned behavior—the tapes running continuously in our heads. In order to change, it needs to re-learn through repetition, trauma, or awakening experiences.
- The conscious mind can reason and change at our will.
- The subconscious sees, hears, smells, and senses everything in our environment all the time.
- Our conscious mind can only process what we are focused on at that moment, which is a very small portion of our lives.
- Our emotional reactions are sent to the body from the sub-conscious mind and are messages to our conscious mind.
- Our conscious mind either allows the emotional reactions, or reasons that they are not appropriate or desired and changes them.
- When our conscious mind denies what the subconscious knows to be true, it can cause exaggerated or irrational emotions, or ill health.

An example of the speed and effectiveness of the subconscious mind was pointed out to me years ago when I was camping with friends. We were sitting around the campfire and I got chilly, so I walked the twenty feet to the tent for a sweatshirt. I had to back up to the side of the tiny pup tent to zip it up because a picnic table was in the way. The next thing I knew I was back at the fire and only then did my conscious mind register that I had heard a deep growl. My friends were very concerned and asked what was wrong because I had catapulted over the picnic table (and one of my friends) at a speed they didn't know I was capable of!

I was instantly aware of everything I had done, but my subconscious was so much faster than my conscious mind that it got me out of danger before I was even aware of the danger. Later exploration of footprints showed my heel (as I had backed up) almost stepped on a bear paw. I was suddenly in awe of the subconscious.

This ability to react so much faster than the conscious mind (in combination with its ability to take everything in, remember it, learn from it, and react from what it's learned) gives the subconscious superiority over creating and running our lives. So, it is up to us and our conscious mind to train the subconscious, but, to do that, we have to be aware of what it's doing. That is why paying attention is the first step in getting well (or changing your mood, relationships, job, and life).

An example of the subconscious running our lives happens all the time when we drive. Have you ever gotten through an intersection and mildly panicked because you couldn't remember if the light was green or red? You were daydreaming about your to-do list...who was driving? Your subconscious was doing what it had learned to do and handled it perfectly. (Side-note: This is why new drivers are so dangerous—their subconscious has not learned a lot of driving skills yet. So, the conscious mind has to do it all...it's slower, and it takes a tremendous amount of focus and attention. I believe this is information your teenage driver should know.)

Our bodies become out of balance when our subconscious is telling us one thing and our conscious mind is thinking another. This imbalance can cause either physical or emotional problems. A client had an example of this when she came to me with a rash that would not go away. She had tried everything the doctors suggested and nothing helped. The skin is controlled by the lung and large intestine energy. When those energies are out of balance, it usually has something to do with guilt or grief. So, we followed those threads with my Yea-but questioning and discovered she did not value "rest" as much as she valued "doing," and she felt guilty if she was not being productive. (There is more on the threads and the Yea-but method in Chapter 5.)

She will always be the type A personality, but her subconscious attempt to tell her consciousness that her "rest and relaxation" was not as important as her "doing something" was keeping her body out of balance. She was denying the validity of the opposite of what she cherished. She immediately was able to really feel that "rest" was just as important as "do," even though she will always lean towards the doing. It was about respecting the opposite point of view. This in turn brought her conscious and subconscious into alignment with each other, and her rash was gone in a few days. Ta-da. Resolved in one session by making sure her conscious and subconscious were thinking the same thing. Sometimes healing can happen quickly.

Back to Jessie's story ☞

It had been a month (we were into May), and Jessie's muscle struc-
ture was continuing to improve. The energy flow through them was
also improving, but she was still not sensing any improvement in her
pain levels. This was her report to me from the weeks following her
last session: "I am extra clumsy this week; can't do my yoga tape; low
back pain is worse; the clavicle area is really aching; the pain in my
neck switched to the right during the week then to the back of my
neck, and it radiated both up and down from there." Her pain level
had been hovering around 7 and was still that way when she came in.
Her frustration was obvious as well as stated clearly.

I decided a relaxing massage with energy and muscle work to loosen
her neck was needed the most, and while I was doing that, I threw in
a dose of good-old-fashion, cheerleading type encouragement. When
Jessie left she said her pain level dropped to 4 or 5 and her frustration
had given in to hope.

I needed to find the cause of the conflict between better muscles,
but same pain. Is she simply not noticing the difference because some
of the pain is still there? Is she expecting it, so she is re-creating it every
day? Are the muscles not the primary cause of pain (could it be nerve
pain, or damaged nerve)? Is there an emotional component holding it
in place that goes beyond the obvious stress? Is it the learned reaction
of the muscles that need stronger retraining? Jessie was very concerned
that it might be nerve pain.

To help find these answers, I gave Jessie the **homework** *of keeping*
a journal about what was going on physically, emotionally, and with
the events in her day-to-day life. A line or two every night or morn-
ing was enough. It was then clear that her progress would be slower
because there were some deeper issues that needed to be addressed.
The journal would help us both track what was going on and notice
the differences over time.

Also, I wanted to get her subconscious working for her instead of against her, so I assigned her the task of posting affirmations around the house. They could be in words, pictures, or symbols that meant "good times," "radiant health," or could illustrate what she was going to do when she felt great. I told her after a few days she would not notice them consciously anymore, but her subconscious would, taking in the higher frequency energy every time.

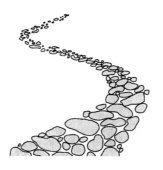

CHAPTER 4
The Grind

This chapter is called "The Grind" because this is the stage of healing when the hard work must be faced, and this is when many people either lose faith that it can work, or get frustrated and choose to give up. So, know that this part can suck; accept it; and keep moving through it. Like Winston Churchill said, "If you're going through hell, keep going!"

Back to Jessie's story ☞

In the next session Jessie was still in the same state as last time, but she had a couple of extras on the list—there was brain fog, and loose bowel movements added to her mix of frustrating symptoms. She had concluded that the enzymes (common brand from the grocery store) may have been the reason for the loose BM's, so she stopped taking them. Again, her frustration was very high, and understandably so.

Both of these added symptoms indicated a more complex issue with the digestive tract. It was possible that the store bought enzymes exaggerated an already existing problem, but it was inconclusive.

Either way, the symptoms were telling me the simple route would not work and we needed to do a full evaluation of the digestive system.

At the start of all this Jessie did not want any essential oils because she is very sensitive to scents and perfumes and she felt they might instigate a migraine. I explained that essential oils were different because they were the "life blood" of the plant and Mother Nature knows what she is doing. If the oils are left as they were created, they contain the balancing components to potential allergens. She accepted this and agreed to small amounts where she could wash it off easily if they caused an adverse reaction.

Jessie's acupressure points were showing a very busy cleanup crew (kidney, liver, spleen) as well as slow moving lymph fluid, so the first step before starting the digestion repair, was to get them all in better shape. Jessie's added frustration and lack of hope were additional indicators that we had to strengthen her cleaning systems before starting any major work. (✍ Cleanup Crew)

*I did light massage (with a drop of an essential oil blend: wintergreen, helichrysum, clove, and peppermint) and acupressure to boost and unblock her cleanup crew, and to move the congested lymph fluid. Her **homework** assignment was to do a lymph exercise to get the lymph moving better, and to fill out the extensive signs and symptoms information so I could start the thorough digestive evaluation.*

Cleanup Crew

Note of caution: It is wise to have a professional check the status of your cleanup crew (kidney, liver, spleen, lymph) BEFORE doing any major work that may dump toxins out of your cells and into your lymph and blood for elimination. This includes emotional work because low frequency emotions are a toxin to cells, which cause them to malfunction, which then promotes more toxic buildup. Any form of releasing, cleansing, detoxing, or raising your frequency can cause the body to start dumping the bad stuff. It might happen quickly, so make sure your cleanup crew is ready for the extra load. Makes sense, yes?

Back to Jessie's Story ☞

Another aspect started to reveal itself in this session. Jessie started to talk about her personal life. She told me about being bullied and teased as a child because she was different. "I had allergies; was chubby; had a deeper voice than anyone else; and I was homely; but by high school things got better."

In my notes, I consolidated another conversation that implied a second, deeper emotion—that being conceited was bad, and that feeling good about yourself when accomplishing something was conceited. She began to cry when we were talking about it. (✍ Why Emotions Matter) (To be honest, in later conversations Jessie did not remember feeling that way, but I'm leaving it in this book because confidence, conceit, and arrogance can be very intermingled in our beliefs, as I will talk about later.)

The tears told me she was hitting on a core issue, and the energy of it was beginning to move. This was a great sign because she told me earlier it was difficult for her to cry, even when a friend died. The fact that Jessie told me at all, meant she was starting to trust me and it was a sign she was willing to go after her emotional issues. It gave me a glimpse of her strength, her resolve, and her willingness to do the hard work. We had been at this for weeks, and she felt worse! Yet, something was telling her to stay the course and she was listening. And then, I too had tears, as I began to realize the incredible woman I had in front of me.

Energy and Why Emotions Matter

The following information is a list of proven facts that need to be understood in order to comprehend how emotions affect our body cells, our health, and our lives:

- **Everything is energy**—there is nothing in the universe that is not energetically constructed, from the chair in your room, to your body, to the stars, to space itself. The vibrational "symphony" of everything determines what it is. Everything is made up of the same energy, but the frequencies and their combinations make it what it is—like an orchestra because it has frequencies (instruments) that create something (a symphony) when they work together. It's the same for our bodies—the many frequencies and their combinations come together to create something (a heart, a liver, a brain, etc.). Each is a different and unique "song." The entire universe is made up this same way.

    Density of physical things is another matter. Basically, the lower the frequency symphony the denser the object. For example, a table is made up of a lower set of frequencies that make it a hard table, while our physical bodies are less dense and therefore, vibrating at higher frequencies. (Note: In the English language, if we are talking about sound or light, then the frequency terms are usually "lower" and "higher." If we are talking about physical density, say a table versus a marshmallow, then the frequency terms are usually "slower" and "faster." So, you will often hear slower and lower to mean the same thing, as well as higher and faster.)

- **Thoughts and emotions are energy**—negative thoughts consist of lower frequencies; positive thoughts consist of higher frequencies. Also, our belief systems are very influential frequencies because they are the tapes in our heads that are constantly running and emitting their particular symphonies whether we're aware of them or not. Think of emotions and beliefs as "energy in motion" (e-motion).

- **Energy affects energy**—even across space and time. The more intense the energy, the more effects on others it can have. For example, there are many studies that prove prayer works. Also, have you ever noticed you may be in a great mood; end up standing in line with a bunch of grumpy people; and your mood is no longer great? Or, you think about calling someone; the phone rings; and it's them? These and many others are examples of energy affecting energy.[13]

- **Likes attract in the energy world** (which is our world). The energy we emit through our thoughts, emotions, beliefs and subconscious tapes (those subtle voices in our heads), attract "like" energies. So, if bad things are happening to us, it is our sign that something is amiss and we need to change course. We need to dig in and find the root attraction affecting us within our thoughts, emotions, and beliefs. If good things are happening, it is our sign that we are sending out high frequency energy streamers, and that we are on the right track.[12]

   Tuning forks can give us a physical example of this. Say you have a number of tuning forks of each note set up so they are free standing. If you ring a C tuning fork, the remaining Cs will vibrate also, but not the others because the Cs all have like resonances.

- **Low frequencies inhibit cell function,** and high frequencies enhance their function. The lowest emotional frequency is fear and the highest is unconditional love. Anger, hate, jealousy, and judgment are all low, while gratitude, compassion, joy, and trust are high. This means moving our lower frequency emotions to higher frequencies is crucial to our health. Also, environmental contaminants and poisons have low frequency energies that affect our cells which is another reason to avoid them.[5]

- **Emotions are stored in our DNA**—and they are handed down from generation to generation. People receiving organ transplants may even experience new emotions as their body integrates the DNA of another person. This wonder in our DNA means that some of the emotions we need to dig out and release my not be our own...they could be our ancestor's (or in the latter example, a donor's).[17]

- **Different areas of the body store different emotions**— Because each part of the body has a different function, they each have a different symphony that defines it (as said above). And, because likes attract in the energy world, each definable body part will attract a different type of emotion that may end up being stored there. For example, worry is stored in the stomach, anger in the liver, and fear in the kidneys. So if you are having kidney trouble, look at what your fears are, and vice-versa, if you are going through a time of fear, be extra nourishing to your kidneys to prevent problems.[6, 26]

- **Our emotions, thoughts and beliefs are the blue print for our DNA.** The structure of the DNA is fixed at conception, but what is "turned on" and "turned off" within that structure depends on the energy in and around it. This means we can alter the creation of new cells by changing our thoughts, for the better (high frequencies) or for the worse (low frequencies). Want to heal your liver? The allopathic answer is to look at the environmental toxins such as alcohol, drugs, or artificial sweeteners, but you should also look at releasing your anger and frustration and replacing it with compassion.[17]

Back to Jessie's story ☞

We were then well into May. I had collected the information I needed to do the digestion assessment, and the results were as expected—Jessie was eating enough proteins but not digesting them properly, and the sluggish lymph was confirmed. So she started on a different full spectrum enzyme that I trusted because her cleanup crew was not ready yet for those that would target her specific issues (proteins and stomach lining). Remember, she had chronic heartburn, had been on antacids for years, and antacids mess up the digestion of proteins. All the pieces of this particular puzzle fit nicely. (I love it when everything points in the same direction!)

Jessie, however, had a terrible week. To quote, "It's worse again: couldn't coordinate the lymph exercise; my neck pain is worse; the shoulder pain is going into my arm now; my low back is worse again; and I couldn't do anything right!!! I let everything bother me…no positive thinking at all. Way. Too. Much. Pain! Every movement was excruciating! Monday I had a migraine all day and night. Such a horrible week I almost didn't come." And on top of all that, she was switching cholesterol medications and the new one gave her a rash.

Jessie said her emotions were all over the place and she was very upset with herself for not giving good enough answers to the people where she volunteered, so she decided she should quit and concentrate on getting well. For Jessie, this was a big deal, because she was putting her own well-being ahead of her feelings of obligation and her tendency to please others. This marked a change in her thought patterns.

Alrighty then. There was so much going on I was not sure at first how to best help Jessie that day. We were a month into it. Was this a healing crisis? (✍ Healing Crisis) It was even clearer that emotions had everything to do with her pain (she had an emotional week and the pain was worse). I sensed she felt what she was going through emotionally was somehow "wrong." I concluded that just talking would be best—I listened, let her get her frustrations out, and validated that she had every right to feel that way. It was perfectly normal and healthy, and she was not going off the deep end.

Since anger and frustration are higher frequencies than depression or despair, and considering she had been on antidepressant medications for years, I was glad to see some frustration showing itself. It meant she was starting to feel the buried emotions, and her overall frequency was rising. After all, not only our bodies, but the universe as well, talks to us via our emotions, so I reminded Jessie that her anger and frustration were messages.

So what was all of this telling her? The obvious answer is she needs to change her reaction to stress in order to get rid of the pain, but what exactly where her reactions and how did they develop and become so strong?

For **homework** *I showed Jessie the meridian tapping technique (also known as EFT or tapping[24]), so she would have a physical thing to do when she felt the anger and frustration coming on. Tapping on certain acupressure points helps calm, distracts the mind from the downward spiral by providing a physical task to think about, and helps reveal and release the underlying cause of the emotion.*

Healing Crisis

The term "healing crisis" sounds like an oxymoron. What does it mean? Well, sometimes things get worse before they get better. There are two reasons for this:

First, your body has worked hard to make adjustments to what you have thrown at it so far, and for physical issues, it will try hard to keep the status quo. The devil you know is better than the devil you don't according to your body.

Our subconscious does the same thing. Remember, I talked earlier about the subconscious being learned behavior. Well what it learns it wants to keep doing, so it will work hard to keep doing it, even if that means sabotaging progress. We want to do better, but at the same time, we resist change (sound familiar?). Anger, frustration, depression, avoidance, or procrastination may simply be our resistance to change. It is very common for these feelings to come ahead of any cathartic change. For example, you may like going to your therapy sessions, but THIS time, you are doing anything to avoid going and suddenly you hate your therapist. GO to the session, because you are probably on the verge of a major breakthrough that your body is aware of, but your mind is not.

The second reason for a healing crisis may be toxins, as already mentioned in the "Cleanup Crew" section. When the body starts to heal, it dumps toxins from the cells into the interstitial tissue where they are picked up by the lymph and blood and carried to the cleanup crew for elimination. This often puts an extra strain on our body and it manifests in various ways such as fatigue, frequent urination, cold symptoms, heightened allergies, bad taste or smelly breath, different bowel movements, or a rash. These are all signs the body is getting rid of what does not belong (in any way it can release it). Too much "healing" too fast can push this process over the edge and you feel like—okay, I'll say it—crap.

Discerning a healing crisis from the messages of "wrong direction, change course" is one of the most confusing parts of holistic care. Is it a healing crisis or is what I'm doing wrong for me? Do I want to cancel the appointment because I'm avoiding the hard stuff, or is it truly in my best interest to not go? These are tough questions that can be hard to answer and they require well developed discernment. I suggest you list the reasons for changing direction and the reasons for not changing direction, then take a break and do something else for awhile to get your mind off it. What does the list say when you return to it? Are there only emotional reasons listed for changing direction with no substance behind them, or are there solid practical reasons listed? If you recognize that the pull to change direction MAY be a pending healing breakthrough, that is half the battle in developing your discernment.

Back to Jessie's story ☞

Scheduling our appointments was difficult for a few weeks so we had some phone conversations over a number of days to keep things going. Jessie was doing better and reported having some great days in spite of the pain still being at a 6 to 7 level, and in spite of tripping and falling and bruising her hip. She had been doing the lymph exercises to get the fluid moving better. She also had been trying out the meridian tapping when feeling anxious, and she felt it was working well. (I took note—her pain was the same, but she was doing better. Hmmm. YES! She was starting to think differently about the pain. Oh, this was good.)

A few days later she was struggling with her computer, and her anxiety shot up. Her words, "I couldn't do it! I actually felt sorry for myself. This mood started Sunday and lasted until Wednesday! Four days! Train my mind for positive thinking? How do I DO that?!"

Jessie was now clearly recognizing WHEN she needed to change her way of thinking. Another very good sign of progress.

I explained it was not an overnight process and I thought she was doing great. After all, she had 70 years of training her mind to react a certain way, and she had begun the "retraining" a mere six weeks ago. I said, "This is not only a new and foreign way to think, but the tools to 'get there' are also new and foreign. Meditation? Affirmations? Positive thinking? Tapping? Acupressure? Diet changes? Exercises? Massage? Yes. All new. So cut yourself some slack, because you're in the middle of the hard part."

The hard part continued with another migraine that lasted two and a half days. "I don't deserve pain like this," she said with anguish. "It feels like a demon is after me—a spirit inside is stifling me and pushing me down. I feel guilty for feeling this way, but I have no chance between events to relax and get rid of this anxiety." She was holding back tears.

I asked about the events, so I could better understand the anxiety triggers. They all turned out to be of similar seriousness to the computer problems a few days before—gardening and trimming needing to get done and obligations to friends. I was beginning to see that what most people would consider minor and incidental were mountains to climb for Jessie. We decided to do a tapping session together over the phone to see if the reasons behind the "making mountains out of molehills" would reveal themselves.

The issues that Jessie brought up during the tapping session were some big ones!

- After her divorce, she was taking care of herself for the first time.
- After her father died, it was scary being on her own, and she missed him.
- Her brother was dependent on her and a constant challenge.
- She was feeling sorry for herself for having such burdens and feeling guilty about that.

My intent for the questioning that followed was to uncover the pathways (threads) to any issues she might have had concerning guilt and obligation to others. I was sensing these emotions were a trigger *for the exaggerated reactions to incidental problems. The session turned to Jessie's religious beliefs. She stated she trusted God, and she trusted herself. She did not feel generally guilty. She did not feel like a "subordinate" to others.*

Let's suffice it to say, every question I asked turned out to be a dead end. I was struggling to find the right threads that would take us to an underlying emotional cause for the guilt and attempting to get my thoughts in synch with hers. I was feeling inadequate in those moments to find what could help her. When I realized that, I knew I needed to regroup and get my act together, because I was following my brain and not my intuition and heart. Jessie was fading also, so it was time to end this phone session with some casual uplifting conversation.

Five days later we had an in-person session. Jessie asked me if she could ask a question. I thought, "She's asking my permission, so this must be hard for her to say," and I did the best I could to help her feel comfortable in asking or stating anything she wanted...there would be no judgment from me. Well, what she said took me by such surprise that I cannot say for sure that I really did react without judgment.

She asked if I was mad at her.

Huh? (Yep, instant judgment of myself. "Oh my...what did I do!?")

After a bit of throat clearing to buy myself a few seconds, I responded, in what I hoped was an even tone, "Um, of course not. Why do you ask?"

She went on to tell me that in our last phone session, it sounded like I was upset with her because she wasn't giving me the right answers.

Oh.

My mind was whirling.

And then, I remembered that I WAS frustrated...with myself, not her. I explained as much and the energy between us soon smoothed out as she understood that I was the one who had messed up, not her. There was much I learned from this:

- *I let my own emotions show in a session.*
- *When I did recognize my emotions had intruded, I did not tell my client about them so it would be clear to her what was happening.*
- *Jessie is honest, brave and true to herself to have asked me, and I was very grateful for that. She could have just quit instead...many people would have. I felt very proud of her for her courage.*
- *Jessie sat with the feeling for days before she asked, which told me she needs processing time before addressing what may be construed as a confrontation.*
- *This was additional information for me about Jessie's sensitivities, intuitive abilities, and ways of interpreting conversations.*

All duly noted!

With that resolved, we continued with the session. She had some stress over her cat in the morning, so she was already at a pain level of 7 (again, higher stress caused higher pain). I had not worked very much on the physical issues in a few weeks, so massage and acupressure were in order. I was able to get her levels down to 4 or 5 by working with all the muscles attached to the shoulder blade and unblocking the gall bladder meridian through the hip, which also flows through the top of the shoulder.

She told me during the week her pain level had gotten to a 10 due to the cat and her obligations to help a neighbor (and I'm sure her thoughts about me as well, but she was polite and did not say that). She did some tapping on her own and was able to function again. Since that word "obligation" came up again, I asked her about it. She said, *"It was impressed upon me to take care of my brother. As a child I sensed it, and as an adult my mother instilled it further."* She also added that her dad died more than 10 years ago. Then her mom got sick, and it seemed like she had no time to mourn her dad's death… no rest between catastrophes. All of this ate away at her confidence level of handling everything on her own.

She had said it before, but throughout the session she repeated many times, "I'm a hard nut to crack." (✐ What we say matters) I gave her a homework assignment to start the process of changing her thinking habits to something more productive: when she feels anxious about something, remind herself that she knows she can do it because she's done it before and it's just another adventure. Trust and adventure, instead of fear and "I can't." Part of this was to take note when she told herself, "I'm a hard nut to crack," then say, "Cancel that! I make changes easily."

What We Say Matters

We manifest our lives (and our bodies) through our thoughts and our beliefs. What we SAY is a reflection of both of those, so changing what we say can help greatly in changing our thoughts and our beliefs and, therefore, changing our lives and our bodies.

For example, when we ask, "What is the matter?" we are really asking, "What are you changing from thought into matter?" (I know! It's a lot to think about.)

Here is an example of how we can inadvertently manifest our ailments. I had a client in her twenties who was having odd heart issues. Her brain was not communicating with her heart properly. Her doctors were doing their thing to help the physical symptoms and she was coming to me to investigate any emotional issues that might have been contributing. What we uncovered was a statement her mother said to her often when she was a child, "You'd forget your head if it weren't attached!" In my client's child mind, every time this was said to her, she pictured her actual head being detached from her body. Because there was often an emotion involved (such as shame for forgetting), this image was driven into deep storage and the body was slowly manifesting a detached head years later.

This sounds way too bizarre I know! I could not believe that our thoughts could be that powerful until I saw it happen over and over again. Once you are aware of this fact you start to see it in anyone you are reasonably close with…they are becoming what they say and believe.

And not only what we say, but the written word, also has power. This has been proven by changing the structure of water with words written on the water bottles. We are more than 60% water, so that means words can change us as well.[16]

- -

CHALLENGE

For a week, notice when you have a firm belief about something and question it…write down your findings. Our beliefs can equate to the tape running in our heads all the time. What is your tape saying? I will get sick when I get old? I can't do this? Life is hard? Rich people are greedy (so therefore, I don't want to be rich)? I'm not worthy of that? Remember, you do not have to be consciously thinking about the tape for it to be running and having its effect. Anyway, you get the idea.

- -

Back to Jessie's story ☞

We were then into June, and Jessie's pain was around 4 after her last session. She was emotionally doing well, and her stress was lower due to not being at the volunteer office. However, that day she was pessimistic after having a migraine the day before. Her comments were, "It feels like my body won't let the energy in. I feel strange telling you, but it's like there is an evil spirit around me sometimes. I tell it to go away (demand it), but it comes back."

This was the second time Jessie had mentioned this, so it needed to be addressed. I asked if she wanted my opinion and she genuinely did, so we went into the next bizarre realm of evil spirits, entities and energy cords. We talked for some time until I was sure she was comfortable with her suspicions being verified. (✍ Pesky Energy and Spirits)

She had only mentioned her brother in passing, but there was more to that story. I suspected he might somehow be at the core of her "evil spirit" feelings. I asked a few questions to plant the seeds for future cultivation, but the time to address her brother had not arrived.

Pesky Energy and Spirits

This is a subject that is not talked about often, or at all. So if it is too weird for you, just skip this section. But wait! Is there a small part of you that is curious? That might be your soul tapping on your shoulder saying, "You need to know about this." So, put your grown up pants on and keep reading. I was there before, too—nervous and scared out of my mind when I first started my training in handling the dark energy, but trust me…you will be okay and far better off with knowledge.

Grasp the idea that dark energy, evil spirits, ghosts (both benevolent and not) do exist. All religions around the world acknowledge it (and frankly, it's amazing to me that we all ignore it…especially our allopathic medical system). You do not have to think of evil, or whatever name you give it, as anything other than low frequency energy, because that's exactly what it is: energy in motion that has a low frequency. It may have intelligence or may not. It does not matter because you can treat it all the same way. (Note: this section is about the low frequencies, but the high frequency entities exist also…the only difference is we usually don't mind them being around.)

Remember, likes attract, so the low frequencies that are buzzing around (your body, your house, your office, or the building you just walked into) will attract other low frequencies. When you come across them, you may feel weighted down, feel a bit creepy (and you may shudder as your spine recognizes it), feel a touch of nausea, or feel like getting the heck out of there. We've all been in a place that gives us the creeps and we want to exit quickly…there was low frequency there that did not resonate with us. Being in a low frequency area for long periods of time can lower your own frequency enough that you can become ill, attract injuries or hard times, feel depressed or anxious, or simply feel weighted down.

What I call low frequency energy balls are just what that implies… energy balls that can collect on or in a person or thing. There are video and still cameras (bio-field imaging) that can capture pictures of energy that is beyond our field of vision. I saw one of these videos of a person on meth. You could see hundreds of these low frequency energy balls hanging off this person. His energy picture did not reflect his physical looks anymore and in the video he looked like a zombie, which brings me to the next idea of possession. Yes, that exists too! I know, it's getting really scary now, but stick with me, it will get better.

Low frequency energy that has intelligence can take over a body and the original person occupying it usually has no idea. What can this feel like? Unexplained mood swings, extreme depression or fearfulness (sometimes to the point of suicide), behavior that is not the norm, violence, lapses in memory, and a feeling that you have no control over your thoughts. The word "possession" itself can invoke an emotional reaction, so I prefer the term "hitchhiker" which is less threatening to the subconscious.

(Note: If any of these symptoms are indeed because of hitch-hikers, allopathic medicine always diagnoses them as something else and prescribes pharmaceuticals that make it worse (low frequency entities love to live in and around pharmaceuticals of this nature). Allopathic medicine will continue to drug people into oblivion until it, as an institution, acknowledges that posses-sion is possible and even a very high probability. Yes, I'm being harsh here, but it's time someone points the finger at what is wrong and shouts, "Enough!" Enough of denying what is known around the world to be true. Enough of thinking drugs are the only answer. Enough of locking those in need of spiritual help into a life that is not theirs. Enough of large institutions locking the doctors into a one size fits all practice. The time to wake up and change is now. Nuff said.)

There is a third type of low frequency energy that also needs to be considered...somebody else's. People you know, events you think about, or unsavory neighbors, all have energy cords connected to you and whatever their primary emotions are, they may feel like they're yours, especially if they are low fre-quency and you are empathic. If this is sustained without you recognizing that it's not really yours, the energy balls can follow the cords that lead to you and end up really being yours.

Okay, I've defined three types of pesky energy: low frequency energy balls, low frequency hitchhikers, and other people's low frequency. If you think you have any of them hanging around, you do not need to know which is which, because they all can be handled the same. Why? Because low frequency does not like love. It's the opposite end of the frequency spectrum and they cannot coexist. So send it love and the pesky energy transmutes or moves on. It's the same as turning on a light and the dark disappears…they cannot coexist.

If it's low frequency energy balls being experienced, the physical act of brushing them off and visualizing them being whisked away and disappearing while you are feeling confident and loving will be enough. I had one client who felt weighted down. She felt a great deal lighter and happier after setting her intent to release any low frequencies that were not to her benefit, and simply imagining her feet slipping out of cement blocks. As mentioned above, another way is to use crystals, such as selenite, to use as your "brush" to physically brush your aura clean of pesky energy.

If it's emotional energy that is not yours, you can imagine the cords between you and whomever/whatever being released from you and sent back to them with love and compassion for their hard times.

Remember, this is about raising frequency; so do not go towards aggressive thinking about pesky energy, such as destroying it or despising it. Again, and always, remember to set your intent and think high frequency thoughts of "loving" them away. Imagine them leaving to go to their next highest destination that will help them evolve.

Sounds so simple, right? Well, the concept is, but "sending it love" can be more complex than it seems. A person in the middle of a meth addiction is incapable of "sending it love," so friends, family, and their practitioners will have to help, and keep it up until the person can feel it themselves…this could take a while to say the least. The same for someone depressed…they may not be able to feel love, or any of the higher frequencies like gratitude and compassion. Even though they are not able to feel the higher frequency emotions, they need to clearly set their intent in order for the help of others to be beneficial (the free will thing).

Please understand how difficult it can be to "feel love" when you are in the midst of a low frequency crisis. So if it's you, don't be shy about seeking help from people who know about frequency.

If it's someone you know, understand they will need help and get it for them, because the hitchhiker that may be riding along does not want them to get better and will play games to keep the status quo…to keep their "home." This makes it nearly impossible for the person with the hitchhiker to turn it around themselves.

Also, many times our "love" is accompanied by other emotions that have hooks the low frequencies can hang on to (or leave until you are done ousting them and then come right back). The hooks can be the tapes running in your head, such as "I can't," fear, worry, low confidence, or feeling unworthy or not deserving. Get with a professional and work on your issues if you think you have intelligent pesky energy hanging around.

The hooks can also be physical, such as drugs (street or pharmaceutical), alcohol, vaccines, or poisons (such as pesticides or herbicides). Even some processed foods are low frequency, so get in the habit of giving thanks to your meals before consumption (saying grace)…it really does help. I know a few nurses who write words that mean love on their patients drip bags of chemotherapy to help counteract the side effects.

Electronics also play a big part in distributing low frequencies right to you and your home. Television is particularly good at this because it is hitting two senses, sight and sound, as well as triggering our own low frequencies with all the shoot-em-up-cut-em-up programs. Electronic games can pull us in even further because we become part of the game. News junkies and heavy metal listeners have a continuous stream of low frequencies going right into their bodies. Also, wi-fi's are continuously emitting frequencies that are NOT good for your body. All of these are slowly bringing you down, so it is important to be mindful of your use of them—find the right balance for you by limiting TV, news, cell phones and wi-fi's. For example: It's okay to love horror movies, but do something afterwards to lift your energy back up again (and keep the pesky energy at bay).

You may (and most of us do) have to work to get rid of the emotional, physical, and electronic hooks before the low frequencies will be gone for good, but in the mean time, keep sending the love…if you do that enough, that alone can work. High frequency music also works well. We are all aware that the movie industry uses music to help set our thoughts about the scenes. Major chords induce happier feelings and minor chords induce fear. There is nothing like Yanni, or classical music like Mozart to scatter the low frequencies away. Turn it up loud to shake every molecule of the house…and dance! It's a great way to raise your vibrational symphony and release the pesky energy.

Energy Vampires

This is a good place to explain what energy vampires are. They are not entities or vampires, but they are simply people who are good at stealing your energy to make themselves feel better. We have all met those who dominate the conversation; who can only talk about themselves; who keep asking more and more from you; etc. We may react by turning our attention to something else instead of listening to them; by attempting to replenish our energy with a deep breath sigh; by the desire to get away from them; by physically changing our position to one of protection; and so-on. These reactions are our bodies telling us to strengthen our energy field because someone wants some of it. If we don't, it will end with us feeling exhausted from our encounter with the energy vampire.

They want our energy because of their learned behavior (that is ingrained in their hypothalamus) that drives them to feed their own ego energy by deflating yours. They usually have no idea they are doing this, and they can only do it with your permission.[25]

Say what? We give our permission for this? Yes. Our "permissions" are our issues that allow it. For example: Sally dreads going to parties because she always ends up with a person who will not stop talking. She has no interest in what they have to say and she can't get away from them. For Sally, this happens every time, and she has learned to hate parties. One in particular is going to be at the party she is invited to (I'll call him "Gabby"). Sally arrives at the party with an energy antennae that is shouting, "I can't stand up to people who talk too much…here I am!" Gabby's radar locks right into this energy and he practically meets Sally at the door, because just like in the example of the tuning forks talked about previously, they are "like" frequencies that will balance each other. If Sally gets rid of her fear and learns how to handle the Gabbys of the world, she will stop attracting that type of energy vampire and maybe even enjoy parties again.

Back to Jessie's story ☞

We reviewed Jessie's digestive progress. I palpated the digestion points, and her lymph indicators had improved enough that I felt it was time to go to the next step with the herbs and enzymes—this time to specifically target the protein deficiency and promote the healing of her stomach lining.

Also, this is what came up in our general conversation: "I'm okay with living alone, but this week it's been lonely—this is not a life anymore. My friends are dwindling, and I miss my nephews. There is so much to remember...I don't think I can keep up with all your homework. Maybe I should start going to different events to meet people."

Jessie is getting deeper into depression. (✍ About Antidepressants) The only positive thought she expressed was the notion of finding events to attend to help lift her up and take the place of her missing friends.

Since this session was concentrating on digestion, I noted her comments to deal with in a future session. (✍ Different from Counseling)

About Antidepressants

Allopathic medicine supposes that being depressed is abnormal, so as soon as you show the slightest sign of it, they usually give you drugs to stop it. Hear me when I say, "IT IS NOT ABNORMAL!" In fact it is very normal and a necessary emotion that helps keep us healthy for the long run.

We live in a world of stress and, as mentioned before, sustained stress is very common and very unhealthy. This can, and does, bring on depression. It is our body's message that we need to rest and deal with our emotions. By taking drugs to keep going, we are forcing our already depleted body into continuing its work. It is no different than whipping a tired horse to keep it moving until it drops dead. I have seen countless people whose adrenals and pancreases are so exhausted they can barely function, and our allopathic medicine's answer is to prescribe more drugs to counteract the exhaustion and keep them going.

I cannot tell you how much more difficult it is to help someone get to the core of their emotions when they are on antidepressants or antianxiety drugs. And, by the way, many times it makes the acupressure points appear inactive when they would otherwise show active, making energy assessments difficult as well. From the energy perspective, it's like they've had a lobotomy—they can't feel enough (neither high frequency emotions nor low frequency emotions) to distinguish what it is they are feeling, so following the threads becomes a guessing game. And worse, when they do start to feel something it is the low stuff…depression, sadness, hurt, anguish, etc. They have to be off the medications for quite a while before the good feelings can peek through the haze. That is what makes getting off of them so hard—you have to push through the "turning on" of the low frequency emotions before you will even begin to feel the higher emotions. It's not an easy game to be playing, so don't start if you don't need to.

Does this mean that antidepressant and antianxiety meds have no place? No. There are people that genuinely need them to function. Also, if your house burned down, your dog died, and you lost your job, you may need to take them for a short time to help get you through the necessary work to get back on your feet. But, notice, I said, "short time." Sooner or later you will have to pay the piper; get the rest your body was calling for; and deal with the emotions that this hard time presented. By continuing the meds you are only putting it off and adding to the pile. What you do not deal with gets buried and may eventually manifest as a chronic, physical condition.

Please understand where I am coming from on this—some people need them to live a normal life and others need them for a short period of time, but most do not need them at all. We as a society need to admit they are way over prescribed here in the USA.

Different from Counseling

Let me take a sideline here and answer the question I'm hearing from some of you, "How is this different from counseling or psych therapy?"

I am not a counselor, or psychologist, or psychiatrist. I work with energy, and emotions are energy. The client problems we deal with may be similar, but how I deal with them is very different from allopathic medicine. For example, I look for the connections between the physical, the energetic, and the emotional aspects (and sometimes the spiritual), to see how they affect each other.

Here is an example of how it went with a person who was regularly seeing a chiropractor for chronic knee pain from an old injury. "Chronic" usually means there is an emotional cause, and for knees it can relate to flexibility, which can mean either inflexibility or being too flexible.[6, 26] Sometimes just moving the energy through the knee can release the emotion, and we don't have to know what it is or do anything further.

However, that work did not relieve his pain, so I asked his body questions about where the pain was originating from, by palpating acupressure points and muscles, and following meridian lines. (This is what provides the puzzle pieces that give me enough information so I can translate it into a possible cause.) In his case the origin seemed to be in the hip, so now we have inflexibility combined with a possible fear of moving forward, which is an emotion stored in the hips. So then, I asked, "Where do you think you are being inflexible in regards to moving forward or making changes in your life?" This rang a bell with him and we had our starting point. As he talked about it and felt the emotions, I unblocked and redirected the energy of his physical body so it could react differently, and simply held the love energy to encourage his emotions to move. As a result, he had a marked improvement in his pain and increased range of motion, which his chiropractor noticed on their next visit.

As you can see, this is very different from our ordinary conversational meaning of counseling.

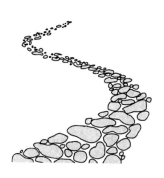

CHAPTER 5

Don't Give Up

Back to Jessie's story ☞

You may have noticed that I had given Jessie the homework of writing a journal and had not mentioned it since. In this session she gave me her first journal entries. Yes!

It did not contain her daily activities or anything about her emotions, but it was still valuable intel:

- *6/2: Pain=8, left neck and shoulder. Feeling anxious...so much to remember! Did tapping.*
- *6/4: Pain=5.*
- *6/8: Pain, Pain, Pain, and more Pain...for the last three days!*
- *6/9: Migraine all day.*
- *6/11: Another headache...are the enzymes causing them? Pain so bad, couldn't enjoy lunch with my friends.*
- *6/12: Still there.*
- *6/13: No improvement whatsoever. How can I stay positive?*
- *6/14: Another headache, had to take Motrin. Not taking all of the new enzymes.*

Yipes. We were over two months into this and Jessie was still experiencing no improvement and felt her depression was worsening. If I saw no change at this point, I would have suggested either I was not the right person for the job or we were completely on the wrong track. However, I did see changes, so I asked Jessie if she was confident in the process or did she have misgivings about continuing the work. She could feel temporary relief after the sessions, which for her was an implication to continue. It was time to do a recap and get us both on the same page:

Recap

The whole process was pretty confusing to Jessie at this point, so we went back to the basics to help straighten it out…back to the four stressors. Remember, in order to help your body heal itself, you need to give it the right nutrition; stop the physical stress; raise the cell frequency; and balance the energy. So was this happening with Jessie? From my perspective, yes. For Jessie, it was too hard to tell.

__Better nutrition:__ Jessie was consistently taking the enzymes at each meal, but had just started taking those that would speed up the healing of her stomach lining. Her body was telling us she was on the right track because her BMs were back to normal and several of the palpation points for digestion were consistently not as active when I checked in the last few sessions.

__Reduced physical stress:__ Jessie's muscles were more pliable and the habit of raising her shoulders to her ears was beginning to lessen. She was just beginning to have longer durations of less pain. (This came out in our conversations, but was not evident in her journal. I took note of the discrepancy, but had not pursued it yet.)

__Higher frequency:__ Some acupressure point indicators had improved, while others remained the same, such as the points the doctors use to diagnose fibromyalgia.

More positive emotions: Emotionally, Jessie was beginning a roller coaster ride of deeper downs and higher ups than what she was used to feeling. For Jessie, this was distressing, but it was telling us her emotions were starting to move and dislodge from their hiding places in the cells…this was a very good thing! But, it was the hardest part for Jessie, as it would be for any client in this phase of healing.

Review of Homework Assignments

Physical:

- *Notice her raised shoulders and relax them. She is doing well at this and she is just beginning to notice they are sometimes already relaxed when she thinks about it…the first signs of it becoming automatic.*
- *Continue stretching her neck and shoulders lightly once a day. She does it, but not every day.*
- *Continue with her yoga DVD 2 to 3 times per week. Does 1–2 times per week.*

Digestion:

- *Digestive enzymes. She is taking them regularly now with meals, and has just started those that will help with the stomach lining.*
- *She's eating more fruits and vegetables and less sugar.*

Emotions and Energy:

- *Notes around the house representing good times. Done, so this is off her plate because her subconscious is now doing the work.*
- *Continue with tapping any time she feels anxious, sad, or depressed. She sees immediate benefit when she does this.*
- *Recognize when thinking negatively. She is doing well with this.*
- *New: When found, cancel the negative thoughts, and replace them with positive thoughts.*
- *New: Add more to her journal entries about how she feels.*

I chose to do some in depth work with her emotions, starting with light fascia work on her neck and shoulders to loosen the tension, relax her mind, and create space for the energy to move. I also checked her cleanup crew points, and they indicated they were handling things well enough to do the work. I asked what her strongest emotion was at this time and her answer was, "Sadness." Usually, I would next ask to go to a place in her mind that was causing the most sadness at the time, but she was off and running already, so I just let her spill whatever came across her mind. (I had to contain my excitement for her because it was clear she now KNEW that the main cause of her pain was emotional...her worry over it being permanent nerve pain was gone. This was a giant leap forward!).

I activated her PSNS (rest and relax) and did a full body massage while she continued talking. Her emotions were randomly popping in, in rapid fire form: nephew not calling for two months...something not right there...what's left after the family is gone but grief and loss?...Christmas Eve by herself for first time...her brother never calls either but expects her to jump at his whim...guilt about her mom's care because she could have done better...guilt about making poor decisions...etc. There was no need at this time to follow the threads of any of these to their deeper meaning. It was enough for her to start whittling at the layers by simply verbalizing them. (✍ Yin and Yang & Deep Core Beliefs)

I also wanted to give Jessie a means to quickly change her spiraling descent into judgment, especially concerning her brother, so I gave her my favorite saying I use often, "It sucks to be them right now." I explained, "This shifts the focus from taking it personally to realizing they are having a difficult time. It is then easier to send compassion and step out of the middle of other people's issues."

We continued until she was feeling relaxed and emotionally neutral. Then we added the positive thoughts of confidence and joy by mentally going to places that gave her those feelings. When going back to the events of grief, sadness, and guilt she remained emotionally neutral, which was an indicator that we had completed what we could for this session. We ended the session with her **homework** *assignment: continue following the threads of the negative and reaffirm the joy through music, positive thoughts, being in nature, grounding, etc. (✍ Following the Threads) Her journal over the days following:*

- **6–16:** *NO HEADACHE today! Good mood all day after Jean's session, pain at 4.*
- **6–17:** *No headache (Thank you Jesus!). Moderate pain in neck with a lot of cracking going on as I move my head around.*
- **6–20:** *Pain is back, worse by night = 8*
- **6–21:** *Pain in both shoulders and left side of neck = 6. Just had an argument on the phone with my brother and pain just increased to 7. It's only 10:45!! He is another major stress factor...pain remained at 8 or 9 all night.*
- **6–22:** *Headache today, most likely from yesterday's argument and eating chocolate. Neck pain at 7. When will it go away?!*

Yin and Yang

Yin and yang represent the opposites in our world. Yang represents aspects such as day, light, the sun, fast, masculine, activity, dry, outward, spirit, hard, and surface. Yin represents their opposites such as, night, dark, the moon, slow, feminine, rest, wet, inward, physical, soft, and deep. These opposing concepts are used to explain how the universe keeps itself in equilibrium.

If something that is yang increases, then its opposite, which is yin, also must increase ("increase" can mean more of, or more intense). As well, the reverse—if something that is yin increases, then its opposite, yang, must also increase. The same for each of them decreasing…their opposite must also. It gets a little confusing because it's the OPPOSITE that is increasing or decreasing to match, which means the yin and yang are becoming more polarized or further apart. Let's take room temperature water as an example of equilibrium between hot and cold. If the hot water (yang) flowing into it increases, then the cold water (being the opposite, yin) flowing into it must also INCREASE to create the equilibrium of room temperature water. If the hot gets hotter, the cold must get colder, thus the yin and yang become more polarized.

A good metaphor for depicting this is a stick with pails hanging off each end—a yoke—one pail representing yin and the other yang. The universe will keep the pails at equal weight so there is always just as much yin in the world as there is yang.

Now let's say something starts to take on more yang aspects so the yang bucket gets heavier. The universe will create more yin so that bucket starts to fill in order to stay the same weight as the yang bucket. The universe keeps the yin and the yang at equal weights in order to keep the whole (as in all of creation) in perfect balance. Yin and yang are VERY dependent on each other and MUST stay in balance. The yoke that one individual is carrying may be way out of balance, but add up all the yin buckets and all the yang buckets from around the world and they will be equal. If this did not happen, we just might just see the time-space continuum collapse. This is the play that we are all characters in.

Deep Core Beliefs

The next concept to understand is the deep core beliefs about yourself, such as worthiness, trust, and power. Deep core beliefs are the ultimate ends of the emotional threads. For example, if you understand who you are (concerning worthiness, trust, and power), then you know yourself well. And, if these beliefs are neutral—as in, you don't have too much (yang) or too little (yin) of any of them—you are an extremely balanced person with few issues in your life and probably very healthy both mentally and physically.

The deep core beliefs turn into issues when they become too much of themselves (yang oriented) or too little of themselves (yin oriented). For example, too much trust can become gullibility, while too little can become paranoia. Too much power can become control issues, while too little can become dependency issues. Too much worthiness can become arrogance, while too little can become feelings of inadequacy. There are many, many issues that we create when our deep core beliefs become out of balance.

If this has happened, then it probably developed at a very young age and you have built your life around it, thus it has infiltrated most every aspect of your life and who you believe you are as a person. The older we are, the more neurological networks (neuronets) our brains have developed that keep reinforcing the deep core beliefs that we have about ourselves, and therefore, reinforcing all the issues it has spawned in our lifetime. This is why getting to the core that is the cause of an illness can be so hard...there are layers and layers built upon it. So, if you are dealing with physical or mental issues that you've had for most of your life, take a good look at the possibility of a deep core issue being the root cause.

Let's take an example of an 80-year-old man who had been abused as a child and was now experiencing Parkinson's Disease (PD). He built his life around protecting himself by constantly attempting to make himself and everything around him perfect, even though his adult life was not abusive. The root emotional issue that can hold PD in place is control,[6, 26] which can be closely related to any of the three deep core beliefs I mentioned. To resolve the PD, he would have to rearrange his entire way of thinking and he had been practicing this perfection aspect of control for 80 years! Abuse creates many emotional imbalances that often affect many deep core beliefs (such as worthiness, trust, and power), which then spawn issues that may seem totally unrelated, but are not. It's a very complex house of cards.

(Warning: For those with PD, it can be very dangerous to do energy work (including emotional work) if you are on dopamine drugs. If you are not yet on them, do your homework about how energy work can help before starting them. If you have already started them, my advice is to work with your doctor to see if it is possible to get off all types of dopamine drugs before starting any kind of energy work. Why? Because energy work has the potential to work fast, which will turn on the production of dopamine within your body and your body will not recognize that there is already a substitute there. This would give you a double dose, which can cause insanity or death. Personally, I will not do anything but standard relaxing massage and help with their digestion if my client is on dopamine drugs. Read more about the study that demonstrated this problem at pdrecovery.org[21])

Egads...this could be quite the challenge for this gentleman! What are his options? Energy medicine could be extremely scary for him because he would most likely have to deal with his need for control through perfection. This could make dealing with PD far easier as an alternative. So he is faced with hard questions. Can he let go of who he has built himself to be and re-create the basis of his thinking (at age 80 is it in him to face that challenge)? Will the allopathic drug protocol give him a reasonable quality of life? What are his support people willing to help him with? He could choose the energetic path, the allopathic path, or both: the holistic path. In this case, he ended up choosing allopathic care, which was a rational and understandable answer for him. Changing beliefs can be hard!...which is why so many people avoid it.

- -

CHALLENGE
- What would your answers be to the above questions?
- How does your yoke look for each of the deep core belief examples?
- What other beliefs do you think may be deep core beliefs?
- Stretch your brain even further, and come up with more issues that the list of deep core beliefs may have split into.
- Then can each of THOSE be split further into opposite aspects? I gave you one already three paragraphs back ("perfection aspect of control").

Now you can begin to imagine how many threads there can be to our emotional health, simply because it begins at conception and builds from there through each person, place, and event we experience.

- -

Following the Threads—The Whys and the Yea-buts

We all feel emotions, but many times we have no idea what their origin is. Remember, the subconscious is the learned behavior that creates our emotional reactions and runs our lives, so if you want to change something in your life, learn how to listen to your subconscious. "Following the threads" is a way of getting at that core tape playing in your head that most of us have trained ourselves to ignore.

There are two basic methods of following the threads: the Whys and the Yea-buts. The outcomes can be quite logical or take you to ideas you could never have imagined. The point is to let whatever pops into your mind be as it is; explore it; contemplate it; and see what pops in next. Never think negative thoughts about it or judge what pops in, such as: "That's not like me"; "I don't do that"; "That's my father, not me"; "Can't be that"; or "That's too bizarre." Low frequency thoughts will stop the flow of energy, so keep it inquisitive and positive. Listen carefully, because it is our natural reaction to ignore something we haven't yet faced. Most of the time we don't even realize there is something new suddenly there in our consciousness. The norm is to start feeling some sort of emotion when you are on the right track. Do NOT run from it—go towards it and allow it to be by remembering: it is just a message

The Why method is asking yourself why you feel this way, listening for the answer, asking why again, getting the answer, ask why again, etc., until the aha moment of knowing you found the misguided thought pattern.

The Yea-but method is to make a statement, then listen to your subconscious. Is it arguing with you? Is it saying, "Yea, that might be true, BUT...."

I know some of you skimmed over this and may not quite understand it yet. LISTEN UP!! This is very important, so read it again and really get what I'm talking about, so the rest of this will make sense. Following the threads is a tool you can use for life to help with health, careers, relationships, happiness, and life itself. It really is important to practice it, even if it feels like nothing is happening, or you don't get any "answers." The answers are more often very subtle, so teach yourself how to listen through practice. If you need help to learn this, get it. We all need help for our tough issues, because, like I've said, we have trained ourselves to ignore the messages. Go back and read it again. Following are three examples to help.

The first example is my own—how I got to the core issue of my attachment to sugar by following the threads. I started out with the Yea-but method. I was quiet and still in between statements to "hear" how I answered myself.

- Statement: "I can easily give up sugar."
- Subconscious: "Yea, but that's a lie and you know it."
- Statement: "I choose to give up sugar."
- Subconscious: "Yea, but you've tried that before and it didn't work."
- Statement: "I want to give up sugar."
- Subconscious: "No you don't"
- Statement: "Hmmm. Part of me does, and part doesn't." (Here, I switched to the Why method.)
- Question: "What part doesn't?"
- Subconscious: "The part that likes the feeling of reward you like so much."
- Question: "Why do I need a reward?"
- Subconscious: "Because you think you're worth it!"

And there it was…a deep core issue…I connected sugar with self worth.

With that, I was flooded with tearful emotion and I knew I was at the end of the thread. Sugar was a way of "fixing" my feelings of unworthiness by telling myself I was worth this decadent treat. As a side note, months later, I had to recognize the opposite was also true—I connected the denial of sugar to a sign of not being worthy. When that connection was realized, my sugar addiction became much easier to handle.

The second example is what I call a "surprise outcome." A client's husband had a boat, and they decided to change its docking place to his cottage, which his kids used also. His adult children ended up using the boat as well and did not care for it to the same standards as she and her husband did. In reality it was her husband's problem to deal with, or not, but she was having difficulty letting the angst and the control about it go, and she couldn't figure out why. While I was giving her a massage (emphasizing relaxation and points for PSNS), our conversation went something like this:

- Me: "Go back to the time when you found the boat a mess and get into the feeling of it."
- Client: "I feel the boat was disrespected and that my husband won't ever stand up to his kids and make some rules about it."
- Me: "Say this statement and let me know what the Yea-buts are: 'I know there is an answer here that is satisfactory to all of us.'"
- Client: "But there isn't one!"
- Me: "Do you feel you and your husband are capable of finding a suitable answer for the both of you?"
- Client: "Yes. It's put the boat in a different place."
- Me: "Let's work on the idea of a solution and not go to an actual solution for now. Do you feel you and your husband can find a solution together?"
- Client: "There is no other solution!"
- Pause

- Me: "Think about manifesting what you want. How do you want the boat scenario to be? Is it something like this: 'I know the boat is well cared for and it's clean when we get there.'?"
- Client: "That will never happen, so forget it."
- Her tension was rising, so I went with it and purposely added to it by raising my voice slightly with this next statement in hopes of moving the energy through where she was stuck, "I know you can manifest well, why won't you give it a try?"
- Client: "Because I know from experience, it won't work!"
- She was clearly getting agitated, so I raised the energy tension another notch: "None of us could possibly know all the different possibilities of good solutions there are in the universe for this boat, so why won't you even try?"
- She yelled back at me, "Because I don't even LIKE the boat!"
- She had shocked us both into silence as we stared at each other taking in what she had just said.
- "I didn't know that," she said as she smiled. The troublesome feelings about the boat were suddenly lifted.

(Note: Raising the tension can help in revealing a thread, but it can also backfire and shut down the path to "getting there." The practitioner needs to be good at reading the energy and weighing the risks.)

The third example is the "not-yours" thread. A client was feeling very depressed and sad for no reason and it was beginning to scare her because it felt like she had no control over what she felt. Nothing was going on in her life to contribute to such feelings. I knew she was gifted in the intuition department, so we just chatted over the phone.

I asked if the feelings were hers. After a short silence she said, "No! What does that mean!?"

I explained, "Simply that you are sensing someone else's feelings, and they are not yours. Now that you know that, follow the threads and see where they take you." If she were not skillfully intuitive, we would have started with some Yea-buts.

> She opened her mind to the idea, and a friend of hers popped into her thoughts. She felt the energy of the question, "Is it her?"
>
> Answer, "No."
>
> She asked, "Is it my daughter?"
>
> Answer, again, "No."

Then it popped into her head…it was the new neighbor! She intuitively knew right away that this was the answer. With simply that recognition, the feelings of depression and sadness went away. The fact that she was a talented empath was new information, so we went over some protection and guarding methods for her to use so she could train herself to only feel what would be beneficial for her to know. (✍ Protection)

Protection

As you now know, energy affects energy, and with the world in a state of chaotic change we all need our defenses against any low frequency energy roaming around seeking its match. The best defense is to get your body and mind vibrating at a high enough frequency that there are no matches for a low frequency to hook into. There are few on the planet that can maintain this all the time (I think the number is zero), so what CAN we do to help ourselves through the trouble spots?

It's important to keep improving your skills of discernment of good-for-you energy and bad-for-you energy. Everyone needs to do this as our world creates a brand new reality. Recognize and acknowledge that it may require some extra effort every now and then. Continuously improving yourself is necessary, but may not be enough in certain circumstances, such as a tragic event or coming into contact with an energy vampire (we have all met those that seem to suck the life right out of us).

First, set your intent…stating it clearly so the universe knows precisely what you mean. For example: "My intent is to protect myself and my house from any low frequency that is not for my highest and best, and to gently send it back whence it came." Or, "I am only available for and accept frequencies that are for my highest and best." This is not a combative exercise. Stay in the feeling of love and compassion, so the higher frequencies are set from the get-go.

Use metaphors…they work great. Some examples: imagine a protective cloak made of shimmering light around your aura that reflects back low frequencies (like fear and hate) and lets in higher frequencies (like love and gratitude); give it extra oomph by making it out of mirrors facing outward; put an imaginary grid made of golden threads around your house; or, a laser-like violet light is a great transmuter, so send it through your body and your house by imagining it.

Use crystals[7] or essential oils[11] that are good at repelling or absorbing low frequencies, or those that attract and emanate high frequencies. They work for your body, your house, your office, your car, or your pet.

Stay grounded! It is important to ground yourself whenever you think of it or at least once a day.

And, best of all, is to keep pouring out the unconditional love. If you are emanating love, it will either repel or transmute any low frequency coming your way. Remember that every time you

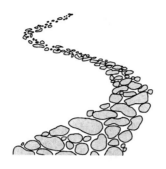

CHAPTER 6
The Roller Coaster

Back to Jessie's story ☞

Not everyone experiences the roller coaster ride of emotions, but most go through some form of it when on the journey of "getting there" from a chronic issue. These emotions have been buried for a long time—ignored or forgotten. They usually surface a layer at a time to be recognized at a rate you can handle. This is what creates the roller coaster ride of ups and downs—feeling great, then feeling depressed or sad, then great again, etc., as each layer surfaces to be released. You may have a more extreme ride if you've been on antidepressants for a long time; if you've been good at denying your emotions; or you've had childhood training to ignore and bury what you feel. Many people find this phase a bit easier than "The Grind" phase because they are feeling the highs as well as the lows...and this keeps giving them glimpses into the end result.

It was good news that Jessie was starting to have wild swings of emotions because she was beginning to feel again...things she had not been able or willing to feel in a long time. In fact, it had been long enough that, by then, most people would have forgotten what it was like to have intense emotions, either good ones or bad ones. That, can be a scary reminder and it was so for Jessie.

This is a glimpse into Jessie's roller coaster ride through July and August:

- *Early-July: Her spirits were better. "I feel good!" she wrote. "I'm actually forgetting about the pain at times." (Yeesss!)*
- *Mid-July: Her journal read, "Will it ever change? There is too much homework...I can't do it all! I'm so discouraged, I'm ready to give up."*
- *End-July: She was beginning to evaluate her life and said, "I have accomplished nothing!" This threw her into a deeper hole.*
- *1st week August: She was feeling much better again and commented, "I know what to expect now. I can do this!"*
- *2nd week-August: Jessie got into another slump that was triggered by worry about what people thought of her—her neighbors, me, etc.*
- *3rd week August: She wrote, "I'm feeling such rage! After Jean's session, I feel blessed and enlightened...even lighter!"*
- *4th week August: Then a friend died and she was back in the hole again.*
- *End-August: "With friends at Six Flags...I had an awesome time."*

It was very clear to Jessie by then that her thought patterns of worry were throwing her into what we now called...The...Rabbit...Hole!

The rabbit hole could suck her in and take her to deeper and deeper dark places. She knew without a doubt that she had to recognize the plunge early enough so she could stop it herself. The sooner she could catch it and start using the tools in her shiny new toolbox, the faster she could get back to level ground and feel happy again.

It's at this stage that many people need a good coach to encourage them to use what they know and do the work. It is way too easy to curl up in a ball and let the rabbit hole take them away. Jessie's strong will and determination helped her through this part. I was so proud of her for her willingness to climb out of the rabbit hole every time she threw herself into it. The old patterns were beginning to break apart. And the best part: with a little help she was able to soar to much higher highs than she had felt in a very long time. One example of this was after a phone conversation. Because she was feeling particularly low, we did a short meditation to relax and lift her spirits. She reported, "After we talked, I left to go to the store and something unusual happened. All the colors outside were brighter—the trees, the sky, the flowers, cars, houses…everything! Also, it all seemed more clear and sharp. I didn't know that how I thought of things would affect how I actually saw things!"

I was quite impressed with Jessie, because many people work for years on their issues and don't experience this type of shift in perception. I believe this happens when we've raised our overall frequency to a higher level, even if it's only for a moment. Way to go, Jessie!

And then, by evening, the pain brought her back to a low again. "Oh well," she said in her journal as the roller coaster ride continued.

I am gentle with clients during the first part of the energy work until they start to experience some emotional highs as well as the lows. This tells me they are through the worst of the initial "emotional turn on" where they can only feel the bad stuff. They also need to have demonstrated that they have a good grasp of the tools for handling the downers. It was time to step up the energy work of raising Jessie's overall frequency. This was because she was now feeling some of the good emotions that had been buried, and, on her own, she was using the tools to handle the downers: recognizing the thought patterns, tapping, meditation, music, affirmations, following the threads, positive thinking, and grounding.

To this end, I gave her the homework assignment of writing down the pros and cons of helping her brother. This is the list she gave me at her next session:

Help My Brother or Not?

NO

1) *He never shows appreciation in a loving way (or, for that matter, in ANY way).*
2) *He causes his own health problems which leads to dire consequences and I'm left to pick up the pieces. This repeats over and over again.*
3) *He has never been a big brother to me. I've always had to be the big sister even though he is older. I could never turn to him for anything.*
4) *He often beat me up when we were children.*
5) *He can still be very mean. He lies and is very critical of others, but cannot, or will not, realize his own faults.*
6) *He cannot be reasoned with.*
7) *He is always suspicious of me and family members (especially me).*
8) *I just don't like being around him.*
9) *I resent him for destroying the home our father built.*

YES

1) *He had a difficult birth and may have had brain damage.*
2) *He was always a slow learner at school.*
3) *He still has the mind of a pre-teen.*
4) *He was beaten up several times as an adolescent.*
5) *Even though most of the time I can't stand him, I still have empathy for him, from when I was a child until now.*
6) *Mom made me promise not to abandon him (she was very ill at the time).*

As you can see, there are many things to work on from this list, but my job is to help with the neck and shoulder pain. To do this I cannot simply think of it as "fibromyalgia" because, as you now know, there is much more to it.

Note: The driving emotion for most fibromyalgia pain is being attached to having the pain, or attachment to being the victim. This is usually in the form of "Who will I be, if I don't have this pain anymore." Other emotional threads may be, "I get more attention when I'm sick," or "I will have to go back to work if the pain goes away." This is not about blaming the victim…remember, these are subconscious emotions and can be very subtle and unknown to the conscious mind. Therefore, it's important to not dismiss them with, "Nah, that's ridiculous…who would ever think THAT?"

That being said, I, myself, dismissed them at first with Jessie, because she was not fitting the "norm" of what I've seen with fibromyalgia clients. She did not at all appear to have victim issues…it seemed far more like worthiness issues. Also, fibromyalgia is often used as a catch-all term when our medical system doesn't know what is really causing it. So, did she really have it? These were questions with no forthcoming hints as to which direction I should go in terms of her next session.

Jessie was recognizing her reactions to her brother were a big part of the problem along with her own tendency to worry too much. The primary issues that were surfacing were anger, boundaries, excessive worry, and lack of confidence. Since the anger was her primary concern today, I thought releasing it should be the intent of the session.

My friend and colleague, Barbara, is an extremely gifted intuitive, and with my strength leaning more towards the physical body and energy systems, we make a great team when we work together. We each seem to strengthen the gifts of the other to result in a more powerful session than when we work alone. I thought Jessie was ready for it, so Barbara joined me for this session via a three-way phone conversation. (✍ Intuition—Universal Energy and Guides)

In the initial chat, Jessie talked of her anger towards her brother for treating her badly and also anger towards her mom for sticking up for him instead of protecting her when she was young. She said she often asked herself, "What is the right thing to do?" This gave Barbara and me enough to start the energy work.

I immediately sensed to disconnect the energetic cords (pesky energy) between Jessie and her brother so she could be freer to make more balanced choices. With the thick, heavy cords that their dependency on each other had built, it would be impossible for Jessie to decide for herself what would be best concerning her brother. Both sides of the same coin (his selfishness and her need to do what was right) were strong magnets pulling each other together—drawing the yin and yang into balance.

I also dissolved all contracts, covenants, promises, oaths, and swearings throughout all times, spaces, and dimensions that were related to caring for others and not for her highest and best. While I was doing the work, I was aware that our guides were very busy helping with related "opposites" out there in other realities: such as humbleness versus confidence; watching versus leadership; control versus subordination; fear versus finding courage and strength; and dominance versus weakness. There was so much yin and yang balancing going on, I didn't even try to keep track of it all. But, when this much happens all at once, it tells me Jessie was ready for this deep work.

In the meantime, Barbara was given an image of a dragon—an angry-at-the-world, fire breathing, resentful dragon. She held the love energy while she focused on different areas of Jessie's body that she was drawn to (the spine and heart, as well as the sacral and root chakras). Slowly, the dragon became a pet dragon, curled up around Jessie, and then it was clear the dragon was there to protect her. This was a beautiful metaphor for Jessie's anger and resentment, as it was moving from an unrecognized beast to what anger really is—a message that something is out of balance and we need to fix it. In Jessie's case, up until now, she was not willing to recognize and acknowledge her anger, because she was "being good" by "doing the right thing." She was unaware that this was showing disrespect to herself.

Now she could define the anger differently as being angry with herself for not standing up to her brother and setting boundaries. As Barbara said to Jessie, "You need to have as much respect and faith in yourself as you do in God to bring your energy back to balance. God cannot do it for you without interfering with free will, so it is up to you to do the work. That's the dragon's message. That's your anger's message. It is your friend and protector if you hear it instead of simply act out its emotion."

After this session, Jessie reported, "The pain in my shoulder and neck is better. I'm relaxed, mellow, and feel lighter. I'm feeling a bit foggy from being so relaxed, but it's like a cloud has lifted." Laughing, she said, "And I have my own pet dragon!"

Her brother ended up in the hospital for a minor issue a few days later. Jessie wrote in her journal, "Here we go again! God help me." She went to the wake of her friend; felt so sad, but could not cry.

Note: Sadness is a higher frequency than anger. Jessie was feeling more anger at that time, but she was progressing and would soon be feeling the sadness enough to cry.

Intuition – Guides, Universal Energy, or Imagination

Intuition is a funny thing. It even scares some people. You can think of it in many ways, but the two most popular are "guides" talking to you, or you have tapped into the "universal energy." Here is where definitions can mess with people's beliefs, so I want you to set aside your beliefs for a few minutes and just get the concept that the different definitions represent. Then you can put your own words to it to help your brain accept the ideas behind the words.

I will start with "guides"—also interpreted as guardian angles, super-consciousness, higher self, ancestors, spirits, saints, or any other name that means helpful beings from the other side. I'll be using the term guides, but feel free to substitute whatever you are comfortable with. The concept is that there are beings out there that are not in a body who help us. They guide us, and give us information and they do this by sending us "energy packets" of concepts that we can interpret. As an example, after Jessie's session I asked Barbara if there was further significance to the dragon. She said, "Oh, I don't know…maybe I was watching too much *Game of Thrones*." I could not stop laughing…that statement was so funny because it represented so much:

- That we often take our intuitive thoughts too seriously;
- That it really MIGHT have been because she was watching *Game of Thrones* and her guides knew the intended concept would get through quickly and easily by using it;
- That it may have been Barbara's way of interpreting the energy packet because of her filters and past experiences;
- And, that it's a great reminder to grasp the concept and not get hung up on the way it was conceived.

You can give five people the same intuitive thought and it may be interpreted five different ways, but the basic concept should be very similar. In Jessie's case it was the concept of using anger as your friend, not your enemy. Try to get that idea across in a game of charades and you'll understand the difficulty in interpreting telecommunicated thoughts and intuition. Can some people intuit in very specific ideas? Yes, but most cannot, so when dealing with mediums and intuitives, stay away from specifics and grasp the general concepts of the messages by interpreting the metaphors.

Also, pay attention to synchronicities over the next few days. If you did not understand the message ask for clarification. Then make sure you pay attention to synchronistic or unusual events, such as a magazine article catches your eye, or a friend tells you something that is unexpected coming from them. As an example, if I stub my toe, I don't think much of it. If I stub it a second time, okay, I'm listening. If I knock it a third time, OKAY, I got the message and I know there is an imbalance of energy that has been trying to get my attention. It's time to look up what emotion is stored in the toe, which in this case concerns "guilt about details in the future."[6, 26]

Those around us will frequently follow the energy streamers sent out by our requests and give us the answers we're looking for. Have you ever told someone something and then thought, "Why did I do that?" or "Where did that come from?" You were probably following their energy streamers and gave them information that led to the answer they needed (providing they were being mindful of clues). To get our attention our guides have to work with what tools are available within the person they are working with (such as symbols we know, learned knowledge, openness, and past experiences).

Our guides often use animals (wild or domestic) to get our attention. One very emotional case of this comes to mind. My three beloved pets died within a few weeks of each other. I was beside myself with grief, and even guilt over what I could have done to prevent their deaths. The pond on my property has always been a peaceful place for me, so I went there to cry out my emotions. I noticed a rock out of place that turned out to be the resident snapping turtle…right there within two feet of me. He stayed, which was very unusual, but even more so, the minnows, fish, and frogs joined him and lined up in front of me—predators and prey, right next to each other, in peace. I have never seen such a phenomenon before or since. Someone helped them do that, which was my message from the other side: all is as it should be. So, if you are paying attention, your guides may start using animals to get a message to you.[4]

The other frequently used term to explain intuition is what I am calling "universal energy." Other names for it are the field, the ethers, the God particle, the matrix, the grid, and for many "God." It is where all knowledge is stored and is accessible to all of us…people, plants, animals, water, rocks, the sun, the moon, stars…everything is connected to this information. Everything IS this information. For me, this gives the phrases "we are all one," and "we are all connected," a much deeper meaning.[13]

Think of telecommunication as energy packets floating around for anyone to catch. They contain the symphony of frequencies we call a thought form. For example if you want a dog to stop barking, picture in your mind the dog sitting contentedly with its mouth closed. Mentally give this image to the dog. The dog (and everyone else) now has the entire symphony of frequencies available that means "be quiet." It is up to him to pay attention to it or not. The energy packet has no language—it is entirely emotional, which is why each person will interpret the intent of the "be quiet" packet in their own language. The information of the entire universe is in the ethers inside these little energy packets. It's like a library full of them—just ask for the information and it's there.

Animals are still very tuned into the universal energy, while we humans have tuned it out and don't listen anymore because of our belief systems. This explains things like yearly animal migration, and why they know to go to higher ground before the tsunami hits and we don't. (Side note: add to that the concept of all time (past, present and future) is happening at the same time and things really get squirrelly, but that's for another book.)

It does not matter if you believe you are being prompted by guides or you are pulling the information from the universal energy, or from yourself from another time. Just pay attention, hear the subtle nudges, practice often, and your faith in your intuition will continue to grow.

Okay, I hear you, "Practice? How?" Answer: "Pretend." Have you ever had a train of thought completely derail and then wonder, "Where did that come from?" It was probably an intuitive thought coming in that you actually sensed. The biggest problem in learning about your own intuition is deciphering between your imagination and a real intuitive thought. The second is learning what type of intuitive you are. Do you feel it, see it, hear it, smell it, or just know it? You can practice and discover both at the same time, by sitting somewhere quiet and opening your senses to everything around you. Feel the chair, smell the air, hear the sounds all around, and see with soft eyes (no particular focus, so you see your full periphery). Ask a question, then let you mind wonder...just a bit. Do you see, hear, smell, think, or feel anything? Practice with your eyes open and closed to find out what works best for you. If your thinking follows a traceable train of thought, then it is probably your imagination. If a thought pops into your head suddenly out of nowhere, then it is probably your intuition. If you see an image in your mind, hear a voice in your head, or suddenly wonder where that smell is coming from, believe it is your intuition. You may not experience any sensory information, but, instead, get a feeling of just knowing what the answer is. While you are practicing, do not doubt or judge yourself or what you receive because that will shut down the energy flow. There is plenty of time for questioning and analysis later. Practice with questions that you can verify and keep track of them. You will find that your ability to beat the statistical odds of being right keeps improving.

Back to Jessie's story ☞

The next session was about setting boundaries. I asked how far Jessie was willing to go to protect herself from her brother's nastiness. She stated she could not abandon him, but she wanted to set the boundaries and she was willing to walk out if he mistreated her again. We established some affirmations to keep repeating to give her courage: "I am just as important as he is," and "I don't owe him my life." She made a plan…the next time she saw him she would tell him very clearly what the ground rules were.

- *He is to ask nicely for her help.*
- *He must show some appreciation, politely.*
- *There will be no swearing or yelling.*
- *He is to make some effort to take better care of the house.*
- *If he oversteps the line, she will simply walk out without a word.*

She followed through on all accounts! She told him. He stepped over the line. She walked out. His response…he is treating her better. ("Yeeesss!")

*Jessie was doing great. Her **homework** was to keep following the threads whenever anything upset her and tap on it, even if it was a minor point. We changed the idea of pain level to comfort level to add a more positive spin to it. As an example, if her pain level is a 7 out of 10, then her comfort level is a 3 out of 10. Also, she is to start noticing* when she is giving her power away or saying degrading things about herself, and rethink her decision (don't judge it, just rethink it). For example, "I'm a hard nut to crack", and "So-and-so is more important than me" needed to be replaced. (✍ Owning Your Own Power)

Next we worked on disconnecting from guilt and obligations. In Jessie's words, "My brother is like a ball and chain around my neck." All of this was related, either directly or remotely, to judgment, so our discussion about it was lengthy. To summarize, Jessie began to realize that she was judging her brother's life when, in fact, no one has any idea why someone else is living their life. Did he agree to this life in order to help Jessie deal with her issues of many-life-times of guilt, obligation, and worry? Is he balancing another reality's karma, so his other self in that reality does not have to? Was his hard birth a mistake and he's living a life that was not planned? Is he here to find his own strength by climbing out of his hole of misery? Did he simply want to experience the opposite of happiness so he could know it better? There are infinite possibilities and no one knows the answer. To think that we do is the epitome of arrogance.

During this session, Jessie was in the process of understanding this and letting go of her judgment of his behavior, and therefore, letting go of her expectations of him. (Note: This alone can release a lot of held anger, because anger often stems from having no control, and judgment often leads to thinking you should have control. Letting go of any of the three related issues (judgment, control, and expectations) can make the house of cards fall all at once, and suddenly the issues you've been working on are gone.) (✍ Emotional House of Cards)

While I was doing the energy work to help solidify Jessie's new way of thinking, an odd thing happened while I grounded her. Instead of a grounding cord, an image of her dancing popped into my head. Like the good energy worker that I am, I ignored it and *asked again for her to be grounded. This time, my guides showed her dancing with the grounding cord flying up and around her neck instead of going into the ground. Okay, they had my attention now. I asked Jessie if there was an incident in her past concerning dancing? And, indeed, there was…the anger towards her mother was coming forth to be dealt with.*

When Jessie was little her mom made her take tap dancing lessons, which Jessie hated. It came recital time and she did NOT want to perform in it. She hated the dress she had to wear and was really angry at her mom for making her do it. On top of all that she fell during her performance (the most embarrassing moment of her life).

I asked her to list the emotions she felt at that time: horrified; embarrassment; humiliation; resentment towards her mother; anger about her homemade dress; afraid to rebel; envy of another dancer who was pretty, thin and danced well; and she felt clumsy, awkward and fat. While she told me all this, I helped her bring it into balance by stimulating the points for PSNS, activating the liver and gallbladder meridians (which is where anger and frustration are stored) and activating the conception vessel meridian (which is where humiliation is stored).

That night, Jessie's journal read, "Went to see Jean and came out of there with almost no pain in my neck and shoulders. What a great feeling!"

Again, "Yeesss!" This is September and it's the first real sign of pain relief since we started in April. I was ecstatic. However, Jessie could not yet see what all the excitement was about, because the relief only lasted for the afternoon.

The roller coaster ride was still free-wheeling.

Owning Your Own Power

There are two sides to owning your own power: acknowledging it and not giving it away. Many people with too much yin energy find it difficult to fess up that they have power—power over their own lives; power to change themselves; power to get healthy; power to influence others; power to NOT be influenced BY others; power to create (abundance, happiness, relationships, jobs…etc); power to protect; and power to love. There are many reasons for why this is: religious teachings; upbringing; beliefs that an individual is insignificant; beliefs that we are subordinate…the list goes on and on.

Having true confidence in yourself is a form of owning your own power. However, if this develops unchecked, it can become unbalanced (too much yang). Confidence without self-evaluation becomes arrogance. So, is there a healthy dose of humbleness along with your confidence? And look at the opposite too (too much yin). Can you own what you are good at without shyness or hiding from it?

- -

CHALLENGE
State out-loud and clearly to a friend what you are good at. How does it feel? Have you done that before? Often enough that it feels comfortable? Are you good at owning up to your mistakes? Was it difficult to say and claim it as true? The answers will give you an idea of where you are in owning your own power.

- -

When we can believe the concepts that we are all of one energy and therefore truly all equal; and that we are not simply "made in the image of God," but "we are a part of God"; then we can begin to claim power over ourselves and our lives. If we can accept that WE have created this reality we live in, then we can begin to accept that WE have the power to change it. This is a bit lofty for this book, so let's bring those same thoughts down to ourselves as each individual:

- We are energy.
- Thoughts are energy and they create us and our environment.
- DNA is turned on or off by our thoughts.
- Energy influences energy.
- Higher frequencies promote better health.
- Like frequencies attract.
- Emotional issues attract their balancing opposite.

Are you still hanging on to the belief you have no power over your life or your circumstance? If so, please read the books in the Reference List.

Okay, giving your power away...that is a bit easier to talk about. You give your power away when you do something against your will, your better judgment, or your desires. It can be a very subtle thing so stay with me. Say your spouse wants to go to the movies, and you don't. On the other hand you don't want to disappoint him, so you say you will go. There is now an energy imbalance between the two of you. If you said you didn't really want to go, and he then explained it was really important to him, you may then WANT to go...for him. This balances the energy for the moment, because there is full disclosure—he knows he is receiving a gift that you genuinely want to give. However, if this type of scenario is always one sided (he never does anything for you) then you eventually stop WANTING to do things for him and the imbalance is back.

It's these small energy imbalances where one is receiving (or taking) more than the other, that can, over time, lead to a failed relationship. We give pieces of ourselves away every time we say yes when we really want to say no. This can lead to deep-seated frustration (or anger and eventually hatred) towards the person or group who has collected more energy than us, when the reality is…we gave it to them and our frustration is with ourselves. (More on this in Chapter 9, *Both Sides of the Control Coin*)

Emotional House of Cards

Often our emotional issues are built one on top of the other like a house of cards. They are added to our lives over time in layers. Most of the time the emotions are released in layers as they were added. It is why we work on our stuff, think it's gone, only for it to arise again later on, and we think, "Again? I dealt with this already!" An example of this can be made with my sugar addiction. There were many layers that I had to keep whittling away at for several years: attachment to being loved; to having fun; to being comforted; as a reward; as a message I was being good; etc. It wasn't until I got to the deep core belief of worthiness that the work made a difference. Having the layers come off slowly can be hard because we are anxious to "get there," but it is easier for our bodies and nervous systems to handle.

However, the emotional layers are built on fragile foundations, just like a house of cards. If the emotional work digs in deep and grabs the foundational card that is holding it all in place, your thoughts, your body, and your nervous system may change very quickly as all the cards fall at once. This is when miracles and spontaneous healings can happen.

Most of the time we are ready for it and it all feels wonderful— like a lightening of the load. However, occasionally someone may not be fully prepared and experience a sudden emotional and/or physical hit. I've seen this happen with clients who send out the intent "I want this over NOW... bring it on!" Our body may be flooded with toxins and show signs of temporary illness, such as a cold. We may feel tired; a flood of sadness; depression; or the opposite—giddiness or manic joy. So be careful of what you wish for or you may trigger a healing crisis. As long as you understand this and do not go into panic about what is happening, the aftermath is usually short lived (from an hour or two, up to a day or two). You may want to reread the *Healing Crisis* section. (Note: If you have had problems with depression or mania in the past, make sure your practitioner is aware of it and knows what to do to take the slower route. You should have help from a professional who knows what you are doing and why you are doing it.)

Back to Jessie's story ☞

September was not an easy month for Jessie. There were many aspects coming up for attention and release, one right after the other. She was doing a really great job of keeping her emotions above the depression crash line as the roller coaster ride continued. This outline of her journal and my notes will give you an idea of what she went through:

- **9–2:** *"My neck is not as stiff. I don't know what is going on, but it's good"*
- **9–3 to 9–13:** *"Neck, back and shoulder pain is back...up and down, up and down."*
- *"Headache now too...this is killing me!"*
- *"There is just no end!"*
- *"Yard work...ache all over, can barely walk."*
- *"Pain and more pain. What gives?"*
- **9–15 to 9–27:** *"I remembered how smart I was in kindergar-*

ten: teacher praised me; a proud moment, but felt empathy for my brother as he struggled to read."

- *"I remembered my parents were so excited when I bought a house. Right after that my brother bought a camper...they were not excited for him...I felt guilty"*
- *"I remembered the pain started when the second cat arrived (a stray). I thought, why did I bring on more responsibility?"*
- *"I'm trying to learn this stuff by reading, but I have to read the same thing over and over before I retain it! Will I ever get to attracting the good!?"*
- *"I worry all the time about taking care of the house by myself. Will they take advantage of me because I'm a woman? A single person is just not as strong as two."*
- *"There's still all these family issues. Now my brother is not being invited to some of the family get-togethers."*
- *"Good session with Jean, and less pain now. I'm more relaxed and it feels like we accomplished a lot. I'm feeling more safe."* (This session was about consciously making decisions to take on burdens or not (it's okay to say no) and releasing the "ball and chain" from her neck.)
- *"Bad headache all day. I must stay positive!"*
- *"Wow. Comfort level is a 5, and stayed that way all day."*
- *"Wow again!" Comfort level a 5 for two days in a row!"*
- *"Too much yard work. Every thing hurts: sciatic, back, groin, neck, shoulders, and head."*
- **9–29 to 10–5:** *"I felt guilty about my divorce because the Church does not approve of it. Dating seemed like breaking the rules, too."*
- *"I'm still so devastated about miscarrying a baby...losing a life is so sad. Was it God's will? Many years later a partial hysterectomy...it was a great trauma."*

- *"I left Jean a message about our next appointment, and she didn't call back for several days. Does she not want to continue?"*
- *"My new neighbor is not very friendly. Does she not like me? Should I try to correct it, or leave it alone?"*

It's now October. You may have noticed from the above list that out of all the possible scenarios, Jessie was more apt to jump to the conclusion that was of lower frequency (judgment and over-responsibility for others). So, this next session we concentrated on releasing these stories of judgment and taking other people's problems on as her own, and replacing them with confidence and trust that she is a good person and doing things "right."

For example, no one knows why the baby didn't make it. It is extremely sad and very tough to get through— I cannot imagine anything worse than losing a child, born or not. But, we do not know why, so judging it as the wrong thing to have happened prolongs the sadness and makes it more difficult to move on. This is where faith and trust come in—faith and trust that it happened as it should, for whatever reason. Know without a doubt that we are energy beings inhabiting a physical body for a very short period of time out of infinity. This goes a long way in lightening our burdens of this lifetime. Shifting thoughts from blame (often self-blame) to trust raises the frequency of our reaction and helps us move through a very difficult time.

Will the sadness of losing a child be gone for the rest of Jessie's life? Probably not. She will most likely feel it strongly every now and then, but the goal is to lessen the pain enough so her life is not disrupted... to have the feelings without judgment of them or of what happened.

When we can let go of our judgment consistently, we begin to realize that it is ALL love behind the scenes of this play we are in. Then the reality of our lives that we have created starts to change.

Another example: blame (self-blame) was Jessie's assumption that I didn't want to continue, while trust would have been thinking I had something going on and would get back to her as soon as I could. Self-blame was assuming her neighbor didn't like her, while trust (and confidence) would have been, "Huh, the neighbor must be having a bad day." Can you feel the difference in the energy of each? Which would you rather put energy towards creating?

In a later conversation she caught herself judging that she was judging! That is a more difficult reaction to recognize, but she did it, corrected it, and got back on track all on her own. ("Yeeesss!")

Next, Jessie really threw me a curve ball and announced she had already started to get off the antidepressant meds.

"WHAT?" I thought to myself, hoping I didn't reveal my surprise.

I was thrilled that she wanted to do this, but the timing was not ideal because she was still having some pretty hard down days. Getting off the meds could make this part of her journey even more of a roller coaster ride, but it was not my place to say anything. She told me she had decided a couple of weeks ago and had talked about how to do it with her doctor. Her doctor was not thrilled that she was doing this either, but agreed.

My thoughts started to come back under control again. After-all, Jessie was on a very low dose; she was making great progress; she was using the tools on her own; she had proven that she could handle the downers; she was beginning to feel the up emotions more often; her energy was stronger; and her diet and digestion were better.

Okay, I got on board with it…she could do this. I did tell her to not be surprised if the roller coaster ride was a bit more wild. She promised she would be working with her doctor and she wanted it over. If that meant a more wild, but shorter ride, she could handle it.

It was only a couple more weeks… and the tears started. Years of not being able to cry were unleashed and she could not stop. Everything and nothing triggered the tears.

Remember, sadness is a higher frequency than anger, so the fact that her anger was much less and the sadness had taken over was a big step in the right direction. This was not depression, but sadness being felt.

I explained that this was a normal reaction to getting off the meds, and if she did not judge the feelings or the tears as "bad," it would go a lot easier and a lot faster. Thinking, "I should not be feeling this way," is a low frequency, and could send her down the rabbit hole faster and deeper. Thinking, "This sucks, but it's okay," would bring her back into balance. Her subconscious knows this sucks, and by saying, "I shouldn't feel this way," denies the very real and valid feelings and could send her body into further confusion and imbalance. (✍ Conscious and Subconscious)

So, she needed to state the obvious, then shut her brain off and not think. This would let her body do what it needed to do to shed the low frequencies…her mind was just along for the ride. Again, this speeds up the process of releasing, because it aligns the conscious and subconscious. No thinking, analyzing, judging, or doing was required. She just needed to trust her body to know what it was doing. That is what would keep her from going too deep into the rabbit hole.

I would like to say that Jessie's roller coaster ride was beginning to subside, but it was not. My job had switched from focusing on her neck and shoulders to helping her get through the next trip of her journey. We had six sessions during this time where I was basically her cheerleader and coach as she worked through the rest of the withdrawal of the meds and the turning on of her buried emotions. Following is another synopsis to give you the flavor of the roller coaster ride that she went through during October and November (the quoted remarks are from Jessie's actual journal):

- **10-9:** A remote session (with Barbara joining us) to clear Jessie's chakras and house. Reaming and steaming, as Barbara put it, to clear all thought patterns that held pain; strengthen her aura and connections to her higher self; release habitual responses and expectations between Jessie and her brother; and replace them with openness, honesty, and curiosity.
- "Fog and headache are gone after work with Jean and Barbara"
- **10-10 to 10-20:** "Throbbing pain in back of neck"
- "No changes. Meditated, but can't seem to connect"
- "No improvement. Hard to stay positive when I'm waking up every day to constant pain."
- A full body massage, emphasizing back, hips, shoulders, neck. Her cleanup crew acupressure points were very active, so lighter work and no emotional work. Homework: change her mindset to "rest is good now" and get as much as her body wants. Picture her muscles relaxing into marshmallows. Continue to catch herself when she judges her own emotions.
- "Contractors working in the house...they are so mean and condescending. Will they take advantage of me because there is no man around? Hard to live with the chaos of disorganization in order to get this done. Too much stress!"
- "I talked to myself, 'It could be worse!' Jean said to think of this as an adventure instead of a problem—a fun challenge. Jean reminded me to look at it from an observer's point of view—take my consciousness up into a tree and watch me from there." (✍ Be the Observer)
- "I'm getting along with my brother now. He needs me so he's being nice."

- *"It's 11:30pm and I'm still awake! Sharp pains in my shoulder blades lasted all day."*

- **10-27 to 11-14:** *Did energy work to help change her reaction to bullying, from withdrawing to strength, power, love, and resolution. Light massage and some percussion (Tui Na) to move energy through pain areas and associated meridians.* **Homework:** *Recognize and catch earlier when you are heading for the rabbit hole, and follow The Rabbit Hole Protocol.*

- *"One disappointment after another with these contractors! I'm angry for being alone."*

- *"I'm starting to stand my ground more. It's hard, but I'm doing it."*

- *"Dear Jean is trying her best to help me. Why won't my body cooperate!?"*

- *"Wow! Comfort level for my neck is a 5!"*

- *"My back is killing me. Feeling so discouraged."*

- *"A bully at the church fund raiser…trying to send her love and compassion, but I'm physically and mentally exhausted."*

- *"Started my day in a good frame of mind. It didn't last… must be a glutton for punishment."*

- *We had a session that was basically reminders and encouragement.*

- **11-15 to 11-30:** *"I'm edgy, frustrated and even swearing."*

- *"Laughing at myself until tears came down my face. Not sure what is so funny."*

- *"Pain is unbearable. I feel like I'm going to die. I can't handle the rabbit hole anymore."*

- *"NO HEADACHE! Yippee. Want to work outside today."*

- *"Over did it. Feel like I'm 90, but I can laugh about it. That's good."*

- *"What does my future hold for me?"*
- *"Unraveled tonight...I think I'm losing my mind. God help me! My poor cats...I'm always screaming at them."*
- *"What is this? I can't stop crying. It feels like all the time...crying."*
- *"Heard politician spreading fear and wanted to tell him, 'STOP IT!'"*
- *"Neck is feeling good this morning. Something good is happening. Is it a breakthrough? Don't want to get too excited."*
- *"Went down the rabbit hole today. It was not good."*
- *"Had fun today. I can safely say something good is happening. I'm feeling grateful."*
- *"Went to lunch with friends when I didn't want to. It was a gift, but I didn't like the restaurant. Now indigestion and headache. My fault—I gave myself away!"*
- *"A day from hell. Tried to meditate. Didn't work. Don't think it helps anyway."*
- *"Such mixed emotions...down, up, angry, frustrated, and now a new one—tired of living, because it feels like a constant struggle. And still crying at every little thing!"*
- *"Feeling guilty because so many others are worse off. Why do I feel this way?"*

What I noticed most throughout these two months was Jessie's tendency to sabotage the good feelings because she could not trust them to stay (like not wanting to get her hopes up for fear of disappointment). Each time I worked her neck and shoulder muscles they were improving; the trigger points were gone; and she was consistently carrying herself in a relaxed manner. Time and again she reported her comfort level as 3 to 5 out of 10, but when I asked how she felt, she said there was very little pain (comfort level around 8). So I asked her why the discrepancy.

Her answer, "I don't want to give it a high number in case it's not true. I don't want to jinx it, and it hasn't been here long enough for me to really believe it yet."

Well, no wonder she couldn't rejoice because of reduced pain—it scared her! And, she didn't really believe it was true.

Once she realized this, her conscious and subconscious aligned and she could be more positive about the ups.

The Rabbit Hole Protocol

1) Relax your body.
2) Expand your aura by imagining it getting bigger as it stays clear and bright.
3) Move your consciousness to your heart.
4) Watch your heart open and expand like a rose.
5) Ask, "How do I resolve this?"
6) Listen and be grateful for the answer.
7) If it is not immediate, be grateful and know that it is coming, then pay attention for the next few days—it will be there.
8) Do something that you already know lifts you up.

Lift Yourself Up Reminders

- Focus on what you want instead of what you don't want!
- Be the observer of the play you are in.
- Play upbeat music.
- Say your affirmations—loudly—with meaning!
- Relax and breeeaaathe.
- Go out and have some fun.
- Make a gratitude list and put it on the fridge.
- Ground yourself to the earth and sun.
- Use essential oils or crystals.

Be the Observer

Taking your consciousness away from any situation immediately reduces the impact of your emotional reaction. An easy way to do this is imagine yourself above it (like up in a tree) and looking down at yourself in the "play," acting out your part. With practice, this can be done in an instant even if you're in a crowd.

This is very useful if you find yourself reacting emotionally to something that has happened and you want to handle it with grace, tact, and professionalism. By removing yourself for the few seconds, it breaks the subconscious reaction and opens your conscious mind to sense what is right and take back control.

Note that this is a conscious means to retrain your subconscious to react in a more appropriate way. It is not a way to escape facing your feelings. For this to work you must acknowledge and accept that you are reacting in a way you do not want to, and decide to change it. Using this technique to avoid emotions will only cause you to separate from your emotions (disassociate) and become what we used to call a space cadet.

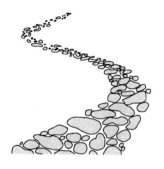

CHAPTER 7
Finally, Relief!

Back to Jessie's story ☞

It was December 1st. Jessie's ups were higher, more frequent, and lasting longer. Her downs had not improved, but it felt more and more like her subconscious was getting nervous over pending changes and was opting for status quo (as mentioned earlier this is a common phenomenon). She was recognizing issues well, and pulling herself out of the rabbit hole more frequently without help.

Jessie was ready for another deep session, and, again, Barbara joined me.

When we got Jessie on the phone, she was still being reactive (triggered) by the lunch she attended when she didn't want to. She felt stuck, frustrated, overwhelmed and had a whopper of a headache.

Barbara suggested breaking the "overwhelm" into parts and deal with each one separately, so it would feel more manageable. She asked what was most prominent in her mind right then.

Jessie answered, "I'm afraid to face the future because I'm not sure if I can take care of myself…the arthritis in my hands has gotten so bad. Is there bad energy in my house? My brother set me in a bad mood with just a phone call. I'm still upset about that lunch."

Jessie's reaction told us that asking questions was not the right approach for today, so we decided to get to work and call Jessie back when we were done. In the meantime she could relax or do something simple around the house.

Barbara and I tuned in and compared notes about what we felt coming from Jessie:

- *Problems had an exaggerated importance, so there was a bigger underlying problem, as yet unknown.*
- *She wanted to be a people pleaser at the expense of herself (giving herself away).*
- *She felt responsible to make others feel better (giving herself away).*
- *And, there was a level of self-reproach when this did not happen.*

These issues were all related, so we labeled them as "The Story" and set our intent that it be resolved and released on all levels, spaces, times, realities, and dimensions. Barbara was immediately drawn to Jessie's brain and the neuronet patterns...she saw a metaphoric image of knotted yarn.

While Barbara was holding the love energy for Jessie's head and upper chakras, I was busy with the lower chakras...there was low frequency energy releasing from the root chakra and Jessie's spleen, pancreas, and liver areas. By the end, the entire left side of her body was clearing and unblocking as well.

We both held the energy; concentrated on the intent; and let her body do what it needed to do with the energy generated. We were sensing very intense emotions and much help from our guides, and what felt like MANY others. So much was happening that it became our job to be the observers; keep the intent in mind; and hold the love frequencies…all the while staying unattached to any particular outcome. As those from the other side joined in and helped, the feeling of love, beauty, and genuine goodness was close to overwhelming, so we knew this was another very deep session. (Note: we do not feel the client's emotions when doing this type of work, because our bodies know they are not ours, but we sense them without taking them on. We do, however, feel the love!)

After regrouping from the intensity of what happened, Barbara and I needed to summarize and get our thoughts together. Barbara had also tuned into Jessie's brain to feel the difference and the knotted yarn metaphor was gone, replaced with neatly ordered neuronets. Her left side and chakras also appeared to be free flowing and aligned. During our discussion it became clear that Jessie's biggest issue was her feeling of obligation to help others feel better. Time to call Jessie back.

We explained "The Story," our intent to release it, and how great the energy felt during the session. We could tell she was not recognizing that her "obligation to help" was actually harmful to herself. The conversation went something like this:

- Barbara: "The idea is to stop pleasing others and start pleasing yourself."
- Jessie: "Well, isn't pleasing others what you're supposed to do? Be kind?"
- Barbara: "You are kind to the deepest part of your soul, so you could not be otherwise. But you also need to be just as kind to yourself."
- Jessie: "I'm not sure what you mean by that."
- Me: "Take the dinner invitation for example. You didn't want to go, but you did anyway. That was not being true (kind) to yourself.
- Jessie: "But if I told them I didn't want to go when it was a gift to me, they would think I was ungrateful."

- *Barbara: "It is okay to graciously decline a gift that is not wanted, especially one that was asking something from you, which a dinner date does…your time and your participation.*
- *Pause*
- *Me: "Let me put it another way. If you asked someone to dinner and they REALLY didn't like the restaurant you had picked, would YOU want them to grin and bear it? Or would you rather they told you (politely) that they would rather go someplace else?"*
- *Jessie: "I'd want to know."*
- *Pause*
- *Me: "One reason you have some fear of living alone is because there is no one to stand up for you. Because YOU don't stand up for you, there truly is no one. If you are not looking out for you and everyone else is looking out for themselves, who is looking out for you? No one. That is creating a vulnerable and scary feeling within you. It can make little problems seem like huge events."*

At this point Barbara seemed to be totally in the flow of energy and figuring out a different way to explain it, so I held the space for the two of them and let it roll.

- *Barbara: "You need to love yourself, more than you love what others think of you. You are a gracious and tactful person. Know that about yourself. Trust that. And do what you know is right for you."*
- *Pause*
- *Barbara: "You were taught by your mother to take care of your brother and she labeled you "the good girl" when you did that. You have learned to define yourself by how you take care of others. This is NOT healthy.*

- *Jessie: "I think I understand what you're saying, but I'm not sure I had the right to refuse to go to the restaurant they picked."*
- *Barbara: "Did you "deserve" to go to one that had made you ill in the past?"*
- *Pause*
- *Barbara: "People need, and want, to know the truth, otherwise, what can we trust? If you had told your friends you were very grateful for the invite, but would prefer a different restaurant, then they would have the opportunity to open their hearts by truly knowing they were giving you something you enjoyed. You denied them of that experience by burying the truth. You lowered the frequency of the entire evening by rejecting truth and accepting frustration."*
- *Jessie: "I hadn't looked at it like that before."*
- *Barbara: "In your mind, it's like people hold a threat over your head of not loving you if you don't put them first. If that is true, then let them go as friends, because you don't need them…they have their own stuff to work on. If it's not true, then stop assuming it is."*
- *Pause*
- *Barbara: "That ball and chain around your neck is there of your own doing. You have the right and the power to change that."*
- *Jessie: "I understand that, but not sure I can DO that."*
- *Pause*
- *Me: "Remember the story you told me about the buck that took a nap in your yard? This was an unusual event, and it gave you great comfort…you cherished it. Deer's message is to be gentle with yourself.[6, 26] Take this all in at a pace that is comfortable and don't get hung up on having to understand this all at once.*

You've had a lot of work done today and these concepts are changes in the way you've been thinking for 70 years. Be gentle with yourself."

It had been a long session and it was becoming clear that Jessie was winding down and becoming less able to take anything else in. So, we ended with some pleasant conversation while Barbara and I simply held relaxing and comforting energy for Jessie.

However, Barbara and I were not done. Jessie did not know Barbara as well as she did me, and Barbara was very concerned she was too blunt and forward with her. I had to admit that I was surprised when Barbara was so direct because that is not her style, but I had tuned into the energy of the conversation and Barbara was clearly "in the zone" and following what the energy guided her to do. We both took a good, hard look at ourselves to make sure our egos had not crept in unnoticed. However, upon tuning in again, it still felt right. It was Jessie's time to "get down to business" and make the hard choices, and she needed a loving shove to get over the fence.

Jessie's journal for that day read, "I poured my heart out. Not sure I like doing that."

The next day, Barbara and I, together, called Jessie to make sure she was okay with the "firmer coaching" she had received. She was fine with it, but had some questions about "giving yourself away," "pleasing others," and "being gentle with yourself." She said she found those concepts intertwining and very confusing (yes, they are!).

During our conversation, it hit me!

There it was—the way her attachment to being the victim had manifested into pain that had been diagnosed as fibromyalgia. All this time I had questioned if it related to "victim" at all in Jessie's case. I had completely dropped the idea in order to follow the threads

to wherever they took us these past eight months. But, here it was...
now...in full view:

**Jessie needed to be the victim who helped others because it was
the right thing to do.**

Wow! It was the "Aha" moment for all three of us. We all felt it
was a major breakthrough.

It is difficult to describe the feeling of "got there," but it is like a
rush of the opposite of adrenaline...for me it's a unique combination
of peaceful and happy. It can be difficult for the practitioner to stay
unattached to the outcome at this point because there is so much
hope that this is the final step (it's hard to stay neutral when there is
so much "happy" running through your veins).

Jessie knew this was a big step but she was not feeling it yet. It is
the norm for us to need time for revelations to meld into the mind,
body, and spirit. It's the body's safety mechanism to give the physical
cells time to adjust to the changed energy and build themselves anew.
It was a big milestone for Jessie, but was it the final layer to her pain?
In our attempt to stay neutral, neither Barbara nor I mentioned how
excited we were for her.

Physically, Jessie continued the roller coaster ride. Life had not
changed for her. A few days later, on December 7th, totally unexpected,
she woke up with NO PAIN! ("YEEESSS!" Will it last? Will it last!?)

We had a session that day in which I checked her shoulder and
neck muscles, digestive indicators, and lymph flow. She was doing
great. I saw her one more time in December...the pain did not return.

The realization came slowly that this may be the end of this road,
but, yes, finally, she had arrived at "there." It was now the time when

Jessie knew for sure, and she shouted from the roof top, "I DID IT!...I GOT THERE!...a joyous day!"

And so, this is the end of my story with Jessie, but it is only the beginning of her story. She said she needs time to regroup and adjust before setting her next goal of "there." If Jessie is like most of us, she will continue to discover other aspects of her life that have been resolved due to this work. She said she will be using her new tools to resolve the arthritis and headaches, and to strengthen her lower back. She also will continue using the enzymes to improve her digestion.

Will the pain be gone forever? Will she have a relapse, or will her ride from here carry her to higher and higher vibrations of comfort and happiness? Only time and her ability to do the work will tell. Jessie showed us she is willing to do what it takes, so I have faith she will triumphantly climb back up from any rabbit hole life throws at her. She knows, if she needs help with her next excursion, I'm here.

I wish her all the best as I am full of gratitude for her sharing this portion of her life with me...and now with you.

Six months later:

A note from Jessie to you: "The pain has not returned and I am optimistic and on a better journey. I have a whole new perspective, and as I continue, it can only get better."

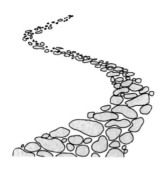

CHAPTER 8
Summary

The goal was to relieve Jessie's pain in her neck, shoulders and upper back. We discovered early on that it was a muscular issue that had an emotional cause. It took eight months, but when the root cause was resolved, the pain was gone within a few days. After a month of no pain Jessie and I concluded the goal had been achieved.

Physical manipulation of muscles, diet changes, enzymes, essential oils, and energy balancing of the meridians and chakras were used throughout the eight months to help the process and provide temporary relief. Jessie now carries her shoulders in a relaxed manner; breathes with her abdomen; has a better diet; and the energy for her cleanup crew, pancreas, and adrenals is flowing better. Also, she no longer needs half her medications—she is no longer taking any antidepressants, acid-reflux, or nerve pain meds.

Her digestion improved enough that the indicators were telling us her cells were getting better nutrition, but we did not follow up with the full healing of her digestion system (specifically the stomach and intestinal lining). She is continuing to take the basic enzymes with meals and this may keep the improvement going without further help...time will tell.

Jessie also reported improvements (not yet resolutions, but she's working on them) in the areas of standing her ground with her brother; incidences and severity of depression (without meds!); ability to handle stressful events; better confidence in herself; and she is finding she laughs more.

There were many cards in Jessie's house of cards of pain that had to fall before we found the core emotion that made it implode and vanish.

Jessie did a remarkable job of staying the course, doing her homework, and using the new tools—even when she was fully in the rabbit hole and wanted to quit. She kept with it, showing me over and over again that she is made of strong stuff! As I mentioned before, this story ends because she accomplished the goal of eliminating the pain in her neck, shoulders and upper back, but HER story has just begun. This process has given her a list of issues to work on when she is ready and she is well enough now to work at a more comfortable pace. At first glance her list looks long, but trust me, we humans are here to experience things, and making a list for any one of us would result in one as long or longer. I've done it and mine is quite lengthy and includes some from Jessie's list as well...does yours? I have crossed out the issue, put them in past tense, and listed their positive counterparts to set the energy for Jessie that they are already history...because words have power:

Jessie's House of Cards List

(You may also want to check Chapter 3, Religions, again)

- ~~Two deep core issues: worthiness and trust~~
  - I am worthy. I trust myself. I trust God. I trust the Universe to provide everything I need.
- ~~Guilt about feeling good when someone else felt bad~~
  - It's okay to feel good. If I do that, it will help lift the person feeling bad.
- ~~Felt not as important as others~~
  - I am important…a child of the Universe, just like everyone else.
- ~~A belief that the emotions she felt were wrong with resulting guilt~~
  - Emotions are my messengers.
- ~~Judgment and jumping to conclusions~~
  - I can choose what is right for me without judgment of others.
- ~~Reactions to stress were often self-defeating~~
  - I react to stress with confidence, and calm action for resolution.
- ~~Fear of living alone~~
  - I have already lived alone and have done well. I can keep doing it.
- ~~Over-reaction to negative events and problems~~
  - I easily see problems as an adventure from which I will learn. I stand up for myself, so I am always here for me.
- ~~Felt guilty if she put herself first~~
  - I put myself first with tact, compassion, and love for all.
- ~~Felt over-burdened~~
  - I know I can handle what comes my way with ease and confidence.

- ~~Obligated to help others~~
  - I like helping others and I do so by joyfully giving without depleting myself.
- ~~A general "I can't" attitude~~
  - I can! I know I can!
- ~~Unexpressed sadness, grief, and anger~~
  - Sadness is part of life. I accept it and let it flow through me.
- ~~Regret of making poor decisions in the past~~
  - I feel regret only long enough to learn from it. Then I release it and move on.
- ~~Expected the pain to continue~~
  - I am grateful for experiencing the pain because it led me to a new path. I got the message and no longer need it, so I set it free.
- ~~Over-worried~~
  - I know worry is a lack of trust. I hear the message and I am following its threads to trust.
- ~~Gave herself away~~
  - I always speak my truth, with compassion, trust, and love in my heart.
- And the corner stone of the house of cards: ~~The perceived requirement to be the victim through obligation to help others to the point of sabotaging herself.~~
  - My obligation is to be true to myself. If I can help others while doing that, I do so joyfully.

All of these issues are related and are renditional twists of the same core beliefs of worthiness and trust…the corner stones of Jessie's house of cards. Each issue had created a layer of low frequency energy. The cumulated effect reduced the capacity of Jessie's cells to function. As each layer was peeled away her frequency inched a bit higher. Eventually that enabled her to pull the core supporting card and the house of cards fell. Her frequency was raised to a level high enough to enable her body to "remember" what it was meant to do.

Her pain was gone!

PART II

GETTING THERE—BEYOND WELLNESS

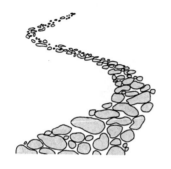

"In a gentle way, you can shake the world."

— Mohandas Gandhi —

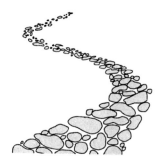

CHAPTER 9

Helping More Than Yourself

What does "beyond wellness" mean? When we are well and balanced, we create high frequency energy within and around us and our environment. That, in turn, sends well and balanced energy streamers into the ethers that fortify the high frequency energy of others doing the same thing from around the world. The same happens in reverse, which is how we got into this mess...too many people fortified the low frequency energies, such as fear and aggression.

The human race tends to think of the more "active" imbalances or aggressive behaviors as generating more undesirable frequencies than their equal counterparts of more "passive" imbalances and compromising behaviors. For example, we tend to think the bully is more "bad" than the wallflower, or the person with an aggressive ego as instigating more problems than a person living in fear. The truth is they are both equally out of balance and both equally generating low frequencies. It is our nurturing instincts that drive us to help the wallflowers and the fearful but condemn the bullies and the aggressors. However, from an energy standpoint they are equal but opposite—yin and yang—both out of balance.

Helping yourself go beyond wellness can take you to higher and higher levels of abundance, knowledge, skills, confidence and sheer joy for life. This is what "the new paradigm" is all about: if you raise yourself, you change your environment; which adds to the change of your community; which adds to the change of your country; and adds to the change of the world. It's about shifting our beliefs from negative thinking to positive, and from out-of-balance thinking to balanced thoughts:

- from "we have to fight for what we want,"
  to "we are powerful and create what we want";
- from "there is not enough so we have to make sure we get our share,"
  to "sharing increases our abundance";
- from "we need to fear those who think differently,"
  to "we are curious about differing points of views and trust there is an answer when we need to come together";
- from "we have no control,"
  to "we create our own reality";
- from "we are not capable,"
  to "we have abilities beyond our imaginations."

The Balance of Wellness

I want to clarify what may seem like conflicting ideas. First, if the information in the *Yin and Yang* section and the *Deep Core Beliefs* section of Chapter 5 is gone from your memory, I advise you to read it again. I said that yin and yang always balance each other...this is the law of the universe and must happen. Our beliefs can get out of balance and become too much of them, or too little of them, which develops "issues", which keep us out of balance.

I also said in the yoke example that yin and yang balance each other by staying the same weight. But, if yin and yang have to stay in balance, how can we create "issues" to begin with? Why don't our beliefs just stay in balance? Answer: Because yin and yang have the entire universe to balance each other...it does not have to happen within you, or your home, or your society, your relationships or your country. However, the balancing energy to your issue is usually close by because yin and yang attract each other when things are amiss...if it's close by, it's coming your way.

But, think of that idea within a whole society, or say a town. Let's say this imaginary town was perfectly balanced in worthiness, and then a person in that town became unbalanced in worthiness by believing he was not smart enough to make decisions. This created an imbalance of too much yin (for fun, I'll call this person Underling). Now the universe has four choices to create balance.

1) Change a person, thing, place, or event to create greater yang within the town.

2) Create the greater yang in another town.

3) Create the greater yang within Underling.

4) Shift Underling's worthiness belief back to balance so there is no need for more yang.

With this example you can see how one person getting off balance can create a chain reaction that goes beyond themselves.

Let me expound upon the idea of this chain reaction with the yoke metaphor to help explain the enormity of this concept. This is not standard Western thinking, so I want you to take your time with this section. I had to re-write it five times to get it as clear as I could, so do not feel bad if you have to read it more than once before it sinks in—consider that the norm.

If everyone in town is well balanced in their worthiness (no one has either too much, or too little), then the yolk has no weight at either end. I'll call this state nirvana.

However, Underling has created an imbalance of too much yin. This adds sand to his yin bucket (he is not in nirvana anymore) AND creates an imbalance between the two ends of his yoke. The universe says, "Can't have that!", so fixes it by attracting someone who is willing to become a "know-it-all" (too much yang) and finds one called Egghead within the town. Egghead's yang bucket gets the balancing amount of sand, so the town as a whole has stayed in balance (the town has equal amounts of sand in all of the cumulative yin and yang buckets).

Yet, Underling and Egghead are both out of balance—they each have two buckets that are not of the same weight, but the sum of the two yin buckets and the sum of the two yang buckets are equal. They are now emotionally tied together because they depend on each other to provide their balancing emotion—Underling needs someone to be smarter than him and Egghead needs someone to be smarter than. Until one of them changes, they are stuck with each other.

When I was a kid, "really bad kids" were the ones who smoked in the bathrooms. Now the "really bad kids" are the ones who use guns and knives against other kids. What has happened? Both the yin and yang emotional imbalances got greater. For every kid wielding a knife, there is another dealing with despair (or the like) so the world stays in homeostasis. In our metaphor, the buckets got a lot heavier and farther away from being empty (meaning nirvana). The world as a whole is still balanced because there is still just as much yin as there is yang, but it is dealing with a much greater potential for more intense emotions because there are a lot of yokes that individuals are carrying that are way out of balance and unstable. For those contributing to this imbalance, they can easily be sent to the extreme of their emotions because they are carrying a load that is easily tipped over. This is what's making the world seem like it's gone crazy.

On the surface, this world craziness may seem like it needs better government to fix it, but deep down it is comprised of belief system imbalances that have spawned a world full of issues. This is why I believe holistic health care is the answer to fixing the craziness. The fix is not going to come from the top down because governments and institutions are immersed in the issues. It's coming from the bottom up; the grass roots; the individuals who see what I have just explained and are working on their stuff.

Let's pretend that Underling gets tired of taking orders from Egghead, and wants to do something about it. There are many choices available to accomplish this. He could walk away and have nothing to do with Egghead anymore. He could kill him, so his problem would be gone along with him. He could lock Egghead up or demand that Egghead be rehabilitated. He could tell the world that Egghead is wrong in an attempt to shame him into giving up his know-it-all attitude, etc., etc. As you can see this is an example of the microcosm having the same issues as the macrocosm. Oh, wait, it's the macrocosm having the same issues as the microcosm. Yes! That's it! ...THE WORLD REFLECTING THE ISSUES OF THE INDIVIDUALS.

The yoke shows us that NONE of these so called solutions will work, because NONE of them either brings the buckets back into balance for Underling, or lessens the weight of the yin bucket by lessening the intensity of his issue. If he were to choose one of those so-called solutions, his problem would only be solved for as long as it takes the universe to send him the balancing yang energy in another form.

So how does Underling get Egghead off his back? He fixes his issue of feeling unworthy. What does this do? It lets sand out of his yin bucket so it is closer to being empty (i.e. he raises his frequency so he is closer to nirvana) and it brings his own balance closer to an even yoke (his worthiness belief becomes balanced so his issue of too much yin disappears).

This is great for Underling, but what does this do about Egghead? After all he is still here! Egghead also has many choices. He's not going to find his balance with Underling anymore, so staying the same is not one of his choices…he must change. He may look for someone else to boss around; he may find it in creation of events that feed his ego; he may create the opposite issue within himself; or he may suddenly understand he has an issue and start working on correcting it. One of these things HAS to happen.

Okay, now let's pretend that there are many Underlings out there in the world, and they all decide to bring their worthiness beliefs back into balance. This leaves the Eggheads with no one out there to help balance their worthiness issues, so it limits their choices to: 1) creating the opposite issue within themselves (which, by the way, would ultimately mean self-destruction), or 2) they could see their imbalance and fix it. They can no longer play the game, because there's no one to play with, and this game needs a partner.

In this pretend scenario, the town becomes balanced again and is sending its energy vibrations out into the universe, that join up with like symphonies already in existence. This strengthens the mass consciousness of worthiness but also eliminates the counter balance for Eggheads…thus they will naturally either balance their belief or self-destruct. Now that you know this, you can see this happening all over the globe. We are slowly emptying the buckets so once again, the really bad kids are the ones that smoke in the bathrooms. The craziness is really coming from the "kids" with too much yang type of imbalances fighting to hang on to their stuff, because it's getting harder and harder for them to do that as more people bring themselves into balance.

Corporations, economic systems, and governments that were built through the imbalance of too much yang are beginning their implosion simply because people around the world are balancing their beliefs. All it takes is for each of us to balance our own beliefs. The Underlings can inherit the earth, not by staying meek, and not by becoming aggressive, but by becoming balanced...then it's game over for the Eggheads.

Energy has no judgment—it just does its job of staying in equilibrium. Our bodies and everything in this world always work their way towards homeostasis. Whether we know we are doing it or not we are creating our world by the choices we make—choices that change the weight of the buckets we are carrying (closer or farther from nirvana). No matter what amount we have chosen to carry, somewhere in the world there exists its balancing weight. This is what is meant by "we create our own reality."

If you want to fix your health, your business, your home, your relationships, or your life, and you don't know what your issues are, then look for what you wish to be gone from your life. (Underling wanted the know-it-all bossiness of Egghead to be gone.) Find its opposite in your environment and you have most likely found one of your issues. (For Underling it was the belief he was not smart enough.) What pushes your buttons? What belief do you have in you that is attracting it? What you want to get rid of is the universe tapping on your head, to let you know there is something amiss. Listen to it, fix it, and your correction will have far-reaching effects beyond your own wellness. For example, you may want to "get rid of" the constant belittling coming from your cousin at every family gathering. Some opposites to "belittle" are praise, encouragement, or admiration. You would then ask yourself some questions. Do you lack those in your life? Do you tell yourself you don't deserve encouragement? Do you feel "little" in anyway?

- -

CHALLENGE

This challenge will create a list of beliefs that, if you continue the work to change them, will rock your world towards happiness, wellness, and abundance.

- Make a list of what pushes your buttons (like what people say or actions that upset you). Beside each item, list the possible opposites. Which ones on the "opposite list" do you resonate with as your own issues?
- Make a list of what pushes your family members' buttons, and list any opposite emotions you can think of for each. Are any of them your issues that are contributing to the problem?
- Make a list of your own attributes that you do not like. Alongside of it write their possible opposites.
- Do the same for your feelings of lack or scarcity, and the same for excess.

Remember that our issues can come from other lifetimes or ancestors' DNA, so you may not relate to them. For this reason, it's a good idea to work on all of the "opposite" items you listed. My suggestion is to pick one at a time and start with meridian tapping.[24]

- -

Both Sides of the Control Coin

If we could solve the control issues of the world, all the problems would be gone. Well, almost all…the rest could be resolved easily if none of us were trying to control the others. You can see the effects of out-of-balance-control in all aspects of our lives, from the macrocosm of the world to the microcosms of each individual. Most people on the planet have some aspect of control as one of their big emotional issues. So what are the different aspects? How does control manifest and what are the triggers? As you read further about the different aspects, keep in mind what may be different sides of the same coin, because for every emotional issue there is its opposite. As mentioned above, neither can exist without the other.

Being over-controlled as a child (i.e. being told what to do all the time, and not being allowed to make age appropriate decisions) can manifest into the child dreaming that they can one day be that person in control. So, when they are an adult, they exhibit the same controlling behavior, because to them, being an adult means you are the one to make all the decisions, and if you don't, you are a mere child. These people often end up in high leadership roles.

Being controlled as a child can also manifest into the opposite—the inability to make decisions. Instead of looking at their parents as the example of how to be, they may learn the behavior of being the subordinate, believing that asserting themselves would be an invite to correction, so why bother. This often develops into the "good soldier," content with following others.

Let's take control to another level…abuse. If a child is abused, they may grow up to be the abuser, or they may grow up to have very little self-confidence and be very submissive. They are the opposing sides of the same coin.

Take a look at control from the aspect of criticism. If there has been control in your past through criticism; you may become the ultimate critic and the one that is "always right"; or you may attempt to receive less criticism by developing a fear of speaking your mind…no talking, no doing, no criticism. It may also develop into an attempt to make your world perfect, because if someone criticizes perfection, they are the ones who are wrong.

Even the need to nurture is a form of control. Always giving, in an attempt to control people's opinion of you (you're the good kid).

Now look at control through the means of manipulation, as in, "I smile sweetly while I get you to do it my way." Again, a child brought up with this may be the manipulator as an adult or the person who needs to nurture others. Kids often fall into the trap of "I will be loved if I am good and help mommy," because it's a subconscious way of seeking praise, and balancing the manipulative control. "If I take care of everyone else, I'll be the 'good kid.'" People in this category are more often women because they are more naturally the nurturers and men more naturally the doers (the Venus and Mars thing). Breast cancer can often have its roots in giving too much of yourself away to others in a need to be "the nice gal"…which we call "nice-itis".

Are you beginning to see the pattern that one issue (in this case control) can develop into too much of itself or its opposite… both sides of the same coin? They depend on each other, and one CANNOT exist without the other. If one of the sides changes, the other changes, too. If someone is controlling, but there is no one there that buys into being controlled, it's game over.

This can be taken even further—both sides can manifest in the same person! (I know! It's really getting confusing.) In the above example, a person that has been highly criticized may be both, highly critical of themselves or others AND have a fear of speaking their mind in case they might be wrong. A sign of this is after someone has an idea, they immediately explain why it might not be so. Another example of both sides of the control coin manifesting in the same person is victory and shame—how many soldiers have these opposites battling it out within them? These are the people who usually make great problem solvers because they easily see both sides of any problem, but they may also feel very conflicted within themselves.

You can see how being critical (yang) and fear of speaking (yin) can go hand-in-hand. The same is true for highly critical behaviors (again, yang) and fear of imperfection (yin). And, the same for control freaks (yang) and fear of failing (yin). This list goes on and on in all the various combinations, but when you follow the issues to their core, they are all about one thing…resistance to the control coin. Either side equals the same issue: a deep-seated need to balance an imbalance by attracting the opposite. The universal law of opposites, yin and yang, balancing each other…if one changes the other has to also.

Slavery is the ultimate control over someone. We've all had past lives concerning slavery. It is a huge part of our world history. Is that the root of the world's problems of today? Was slavery over the past half million years what caused such deeply rooted problems… and behaviors…in an entire world?

My answer is, "Yes!" Because out-of-whack control is the basis for so many emotional issues for individuals as well as the world's problems of noncooperation, war, unfairness, and intolerance.

Power and control seem so closely related, but they are quite different. People use control to gain what feels like power to them, but what they don't realize is that kind of power ends when the subordinates find their strength. A truly powerful person does not need to control anything or anyone. So, are the people we label as powerful really that, or are they simply controlling and we are their opposites who allow them to be? You can see this struggle across the globe as we all respond to the changing energies. The women are finding their strength and the men are finding their gentleness. Half the world is shouting war, and the other half is shouting peace. The earth is pushing us and we are pulling her as we help each other bring the world and her people into balance.

If we can all let go of our exaggerated needs that have created imbalances and embrace who we really are and what we are good at, the world would indeed be a better place. Let go of:

- our NEED to control, and just BE good at leading;
- our NEED to be manipulative, and just BE good at managing;
- our NEED to criticize, and just BE good at problem solving;
- our NEED to be perfect, and just BE good at organizing;
- our NEED to be subordinate, and just BE good at doing;
- our NEED to be quiet, and just BE good at listening;
- our NEED to nurture, and just BE good at healthy giving.

We developed our habits and our belief systems—our sides of the coins of who we are—by resisting the control of the ages. Control comes full circle and collapses when we realize that our resistance to who we are IS how we are controlled.

Is someone pushing our buttons? That means we are reacting with our own emotional issues. What coin of control is our psyche under and which side of it are we on? All we have to do is figure this out, change it, and the other side changes, too. It's how we change our level of happiness, our relationships, our world. It's the law of yin and yang…if one changes the other has to also.

- -

CHALLENGE (points to ponder)

- I challenge you to get together with a group of friends and discuss these concepts:
- How do out-of-balance control issues affect your world?
- How does trust become a control issue?
- How does worthiness become a control issue?
- How does respect relate to control, and what is its opposite?
- How does feeling safe relate to control, and what is its opposite?
- What control issues do you see in your community? In yourselves?
- What are their opposites that are keeping them in existence (i.e. what is the yang to the yin and the yin to the yang)?
- Who or what is providing the opposite?
- If the yin is no longer provided, what will happen to the yang?
- What would happen to the yin if the yang was no longer there?

- -

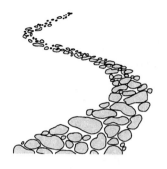

CHAPTER 10
Changing Beliefs

Since our beliefs are what direct our lives, I think they deserve a chapter of their own. We all know that thinking positively is helpful, but it is only half the story. You need to release the negative as well. As you saw in Jessie's story it was a huge part of the process. Think of it as storing your shiny new diamond bracelet on top of a manure pile, and you will want to liberate yourself from the pessimistic vibes before storing your new way of thinking there.

It helps to separate when you are releasing (digging in and getting to the bottom of the issues in your tissues), and when you are creating your world by sticking to the positive. This means: set aside some time to delve into the negative, then set your intent to uncovering and releasing any low frequency emotion that is holding "the problem" in place.

Releasing the Negative

When releasing, you want to get things unstuck and movin'-on-out. If you force positive thinking without recognizing the reality of the negative issues, you may create greater incongruencies between your conscious and subconscious mind, which creates greater imbalances in your mental and physical self. I wrote about the ways to get to the negative thoughts quite extensively in Part I—following the threads, the Whys, the Yea-buts, listening to emotions, etc. This is another part of the story.

What needs to be released?

We all have those negative beliefs hiding within us. If you have not already, start making your list of what you're going to work on. Here are some ideas to get you started:

- Pent up energy that has a "charge" to it: If your body reacts physiologically to an event, the event triggered heightened energy (a "charge")…this energy needs to move through you or it will get stored as pent up energy. The event can be happening in the moment or in the past and just thinking about it causes a reaction. You want your emotional reactions to get your conscious mind's attention, so they can then move through you and not get stuck in the cells. This results in a neutral feeling when you think of the event, so you can react more mindfully and without a "charge" next time.
- Destructive belief systems: such as, "Our bodies deteriorate as we get older," or "I will be ridiculed if I speak my truth."
- Traumas: both big (a serious injury or a death of a loved one); and small (being called a name or a near miss with the car); and everything in between.
- Destructive emotions: such as fears, grudges, jealousies, guilt, anger, frustration, etc.

Released from where?

- Brain: The neuronet patterns.
- Mind: Both conscious and subconscious thoughts.

- DNA: The ancestral cell structure.[5]
- The body cells and organ systems where they are stored.[6, 26]
- History: This life time and all other life times.
- Soul: Leaving pieces of yourself with others by giving yourself away, or collecting pieces of others by taking from them.
- Other realities: All times exist now, and every major decision we make may spin off a different reality...are some of those affecting the one you are in? The ethers are an intricate and complicated tapestry in which each thread affects all the others in ways beyond our capability of understanding. We each are a thread, doing our thing, affecting (and being affected by) the world in ways we are only vaguely aware of. We are all connected to EVERYHING, including other realities.[13, 19]

Levels of behaviors and beliefs

As more people who hold the same belief, the stronger that "belief energy" is in the ethers and the more solidly that reality is created. This ranges from you creating your world within yourself and your house (trivial) to the entire global population creating the world we all live in (mass consciousness).

- Trivial: such as, the toothbrush needs to be on the right side of the sink.
- Personal: such as, thinking all vegetables taste bad.
- Family: such as, it's not okay to eat in front of the television.
- Societal: such as, marriage should be for life.
- Circumstantial: such as, it is okay to kill a bug but not a dog.
- Mass consciousness: such as, we get gray hair when we get older.

One person cannot change a mass consciousness belief, but changes we each make have a ripple effect throughout time and space that may entice others to change…and THAT can change mass consciousness.

Society, history and belief systems

Societies develop and perpetuate certain belief systems, passing those beliefs onto future generations. A belief develops in a way that propels itself on the same track—adopting beliefs that keep it on track and rejecting those that veer from it. This is the cycle which perpetuates beliefs from one generation to the next and helps them become mass consciousness. What you experience you believe. What you believe you teach. What you teach passes on the experience to others and to the next generation.

Experience → believe → teach → experience

Our society calls this phenomenon by several names, such as mass consciousness, peer pressure, and keeping up with the Joneses.

Examples of creating negativity

- Every time you say bad things about yourself, especially if it's prefaced by "I AM."
- Saying, "I can't _____," or "I can, BUT_____."
- Feelings of superiority (judgments, a need to control others).
- Feelings of subordination (guilt, less than, unconscious follower vs choosing to follow).
- Fear of any kind (like fear of hitting a deer with your car).
- Not believing what you're saying (mental sabotage, lying, denial).

Ideas for releasing negative beliefs

- Shake it off (like a duck does whenever it has a confrontation).
- Primal screaming (works on a vibrational level as well as psychological levels).
- Energy work (massage, acupressure/puncture, reiki, cranial/sacral, tapping, etc.).
- Vigorous exercise.
- Follow the energy threads (the Whys and the Yea-buts).
- Admit and be in alignment with what is real and what your truth is.
- Be aware of when you're trapped in your own thinking or emotions.
- Create the space by being the observer.
- Prayer and meditation (ask for help and know it is there).
- The decision to change and unblock the light by facing the pain, the fears, the abyss.
- Notice when your "stuff" takes a hit (i.e. you are reacting in a way that is undesirable to you or to others). Did you simply react instead of thinking or being present? Make the decision to open, face it, learn what it has to discover, and let it move through you. Relax into the hit.
- See a problem as an emotional disturbance and ask, "What inside of me is being disturbed?"
- Do not condemn your emotions. Think of them as messengers, and find out what they are telling you.

How to not store the negative emotions to begin with

- Turn off the violence! (TV shows, video games, etc)

- Be available to experience the emotions, let them move through you by allowing yourself to feel them. Acknowledge them as information, and heed what they are saying.
- Shift your attitude, from "life is doing this to me," to "life is guiding me"; from "this is a problem," to "this is an opportunity."
- Know your own buttons and stop defending them. What makes you angry? What makes you cry? What makes you tense?
- Stop trying so hard and let everyday life give you the nudges towards the collapse of your emotional castle.
- Dare to question our traditional needs for safety, comfort, and control.
- Embrace change because change IS the only constant.
- Be the puppeteer of your life, not the puppet.
- Remain open when your "stuff" takes a hit by not getting involved...this is what staying "centered" is.

- -

CHALLENGE (points to ponder and talk over with friends)
- Thoughts just are...they are neither positive nor negative. What is a thought? Where does it come from? Is it really ours to claim or does everything come from the ethers of all-knowledge?
- The feelings you do not let process through get locked within until you do something about it.
- When should you make something happen and when should you let it happen? Is creating your life different from following God's lead?
- Imagine what it is like to be truly unattached to the outcome.
- Accept the "isness" of the now which will open the path to changing it. (Being the victim of stuck-in-the-mud

versus acceptance and opening up to how to get out of it.) (Eckhart Tolle)[18]

- Bad memories are just thoughts, not reality. Realizing they are just thoughts arising in your mind gives it space so the grip is released and you do not identify with them any longer. Only when you believe they are real, does it have a hold on you. (Eckhart Tolle)[18]
- Guilt. One can only act up to their awareness (consciousness) at the time. Now you are aware of the error and you can then act according to the new awareness. Guilt strengthens ego by keeping you immersed in the past emotion and not in the present. (Eckhart Tolle)[18]
- Guilt serves the purpose of forcing you to look. Once you have done that, there is no purpose for it.
- Our minds can be very melodramatic and can often make chaos where there is none.
- We stay in the playground of our minds and create plays we think are our lives. We have forgotten what is beyond that.

- -

Creating the Positive[22]

What needs to be accomplished?

- Align your energy levels (conscious, subconscious, spirit).
- Know that you create your health, your life, and your world.
- Shift to the belief of infinite possibilities.
- Change the language in which you speak to yourself and think of others.

What can you do to think more positively?

- Begin to recognize your belief systems (be vigilant!), and change those that draw you down.

- Be more aware of when you say something that does not serve you.
  - Cancel the thought, then restate your intention in a positive manner.
  - Recognize what is a limiting thought.
- Find the balance between what you can change and accepting what is.
- Get the low frequencies out of your life...
  - Re-evaluate with a new perspective tv shows, games, relationships, hobbies, friends and obligations.
- Notice when you are not being true to yourself.
  - Are you giving yourself away? Are you speaking your truth?
- Retrain your subconscious with repetition of what you want to be.
  - Clearly define what you want, and imagine it already here.
  - Mantras: Create words that have meaning that you can repeat.
  - Put notes or symbols around the house.
  - Create a vision board or write it down.
  - Make a journal of gratitude.
  - "I Am_____," statements are very powerful creators.
- Meditate about what triggers you to find your issues behind them.
- Do not judge what life brings you—ride the rollercoaster of life with a sense of adventure.
- Find joy of any kind (like dancing for the sheer happiness of it).
- Follow the energy of lightness—go towards things that make you feel lighter, freer, or happier, and away from those that make you feel heavier, confined, or melancholy.
- Feel in your gut what feels like truth or lie.
- Find your faith and trust (in yourself and in life itself).

- -

CHALLENGE (points to ponder and discuss with friends)

- If there is a detour to your plan, imagine all the reasons why that might be a good thing.
- If you're not failing, you're not living, so don't take failure so seriously. Those who succeed are the ones who pick themselves up after failure the fastest.
- Spirit is the part of you that's drawn to hope. (Carolyn Myss)
- Live in consciousness instead of living in the material. (Eckhart Tolle)
- What if everything is just an interesting point of view? (Carolyn Myss)
- Each decision gives us power or takes it away. (Eckhart Tolle)

- -

PART III
WHAT TO DO IF...

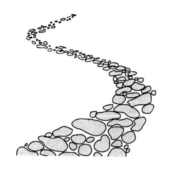

"The five mindfulness trainings: Reverence for life;
Generosity; Sexual Responsibility; Deep Listening
and Loving Speech; and Mindful Consumption."

"If we are a drop of water and we try to get to the ocean
as only an individual drop, we will surely evaporate
along the way. To arrive at the ocean, you must go as a river."

— Thich Nhat Hanh —

I suggest you read all the chapters in Part III, because it is important to understand the different aspects of healthcare from the differing sectors within the system. My intent is to help you see the overall picture of what needs to be done to fix our health care, so you can more easily see how to navigate it. Again, these are my opinions that I am offering you to help launch the necessary discussions that are needed so we can all pull together and make "getting there" a lot easier.

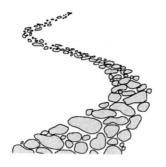

CHAPTER 11
Why, What, How, and Who

Before I get into the "what to do if" answers, you need to know how to pick your health care team, because it is different with holistic care.

The who, what, why, and how of holistic health care can be quite confusing, because in allopathic medicine we are so used to the title of the person telling you what they do. Plus, we've grown up with it, so the why and the how are more widely known. An orthopedist will help you with bones, while the cardiologist will help with the heart—each is neatly separated into body parts and functions—the Newtonian philosophy of divide and conquer.

Holistic care is not that simply organized because we deal with the whole person. We believe the body itself is inseparable, as well as the mind and spirit are inseparable from the body. While there are specialists in holistic care, they can wear many hats if you look at things through the allopathic lens of body parts. So, bear with me while I attempt to make the complex simple.

Like in the rest of this book, start by dividing your care into the four stressors (physical, energetic, emotional, and nutritional).

Review why you need to be looking at each category (just in case your subconscious needs reminding), how that may happen, and who may be able to provide it.

A note about the "who": The name "General Practitioner Doctors" (GP) has morphed into "Primary Care Doctors" (PC). Those that are already including more of the holistic way of looking at their patients, are naturopathic doctors (ND), and osteopathic doctors (DO). Also, "functional medicine" (or IFM for integrated functional medicine) and "integrative medicine" are a "way of practicing," so any licensed practitioner with the additional education may use these terms to describe their methods as more holistic. The names can mean different things to different people at this point in time, so make sure you check with the individual doctor you are interested in to find out what they can and cannot do for you.

Remember, our society is in the midst of change which brings chaos. Rules and regulations have not caught up to the rapid changes and what is now available. And as you can see by the above paragraph, what to call things is also in flux. So, for the most part, you are on your own to fish out the legitimate from the not-so-legitimate practitioners. There are so many modalities out there I could not possibly list them all. However, the concepts behind the practices are all the same:

- Fixing your structure (physical: mechanical and chemical)
- Balancing your energy (energetic: meridians and chakras)
- Raising your frequency (emotional)
- Getting fuel to your cells (nutritional and digestive)

And that is what I want you to take away from this section... how to categorize them, so you know your whole body, mind, and spirit are covered through the practitioners you've chosen.

NOTE!

You read about my expertise in Part I. The following section lists the modalities that are **NOT necessarily my expertise**, but I happen to know they exist and can be legitimate practices. I am providing it to assist you in organizing your path to "getting there" and it is **NOT an endorsement**. So, play loose with this list; know it is **NOT complete** nor in any particular order; and do your own research to find the team you are comfortable with. **Make your own book more complete** by writing in your discoveries. As well, additions that readers let me know about will be posted on my website.

Physical

- **Why do you need to do this?** Accidents, physical injury, or pain of any kind. Note: it is a good idea to have a checkup every other year to make sure your habits are not making your physical body asymmetrical, because this can cause all kinds of problems and pain.
- **What you are fixing?** Skeletal structure and muscle problems (developmental asymmetries, movement, injuries, scar tissue)
- **How is it being fixed?** Through physical manipulation, strengthening, stretching, inflammation reduction and client education of stress producing habits.
- **Who can help?** Chiropractors, massage therapists, physical therapists, DOs, NDs, surgeons, or trainers. Instructors for Ti Chi, Yoga, and other martial arts. Practitioners for ART (active release technique), IFM, cold lasers, kineseology taping, and therapeutic touch.

Energetic

- **Why do you need to do this?** Your physical body is created from your energy field. If it is out of balance or blocked, it will eventually cause a physical problem (it could be tomorrow, or many years away). Scar tissue from past surgeries are notorious for blocking energy.
- **What you are fixing?** Energy blocks and imbalances in the chakras and meridians.
- **How is it being fixed?** By energetically redirecting and moving energy.
- **Who can help?** Acupressurists, acupuncturists, aromatherapists, energy therapists, HBT (heart based therapy), kinesiologists, massage therapists, reiki masters, or shamans. Practitioners of: bioelectromagnetic therapies, cranial sacral, crystal therapy, sound therapy, therapeutic touch, qigong, shiatsu and other martial arts.

Emotional

- **Why do you need to do this?** Cells need to be vibrating at a rate of approximately 62hz to function normally. Low frequency emotions stored within them lower their rate of vibration so they no longer function at their optimum. Raising the frequency of the emotions allows the cell to "remember" its intended symphony of frequencies and therefore begin functioning normally again.
- **What are you fixing?** The lower-than-should-be frequency signature which your body cells are functioning within.
- **How is it being fixed?** By finding and releasing the low frequency emotions and replacing them with high frequency emotions.

- **Who can help?** Acupressurists (or acupuncturists of five element theory or meridian theory), aromatherapists, IFM counselors, IFM psychologists, energy therapists, hypno-therapists, massage therapists, reiki masters, or shamans. Practitioners of bioelectromagnetic therapy, cranial sacral, crystal therapy, EFT (meridian tapping), HBT (heart based therapy), sound therapy, or shiatsu.

Nutritional / Medicinal

- **Why do you need to do this?** Your body cannot run without nutrients. You need to take the right ones in, break them down, absorb them, and eliminate what cannot be used. It is my opinion that if you have digestive problems, it makes recovery from ANY problem harder, because whatever it is cannot get the right nutrients to heal. For digestion it becomes a catch-22, because you need the nutrients to heal the digestion, but you can't get them until your digestion is healed.

- **What are you fixing?** Your intake of food and your digestive system.

- **How is it being fixed?** Methods to determine what is going wrong and what the body needs to heal it. Diet changes, enzymes, or probiotics. Occasionally surgery or medications.

- **Who can help?**
  - For body signs assessments: acupressurists, digestive enzymes specialists. Practitioners of: bioelectromagnetic therapies, kinesiology.
  - For healing: acupressurists, acupuncturists, dieticians, digestive enzymes specialists, energy therapists, DOs, nutritionists, NDs, surgeons. Practitioners of: heart-

based therapy, bioelectromagnetic therapy, IFM, sound therapy.

- **What about medicines?** Holistic care is about using what Mother Nature provides: fresh food, essential oils, herbs, homeopathics, or essences. If you can, choose these first, before pharmaceuticals.

I hope this gives you a means to organize your thinking to better fit with holistic care. Shed the allopathic idea of a "diagnosis" for a "disease"; simply read what your body is telling you; then give it what it wants.

- -

CHALLENGE
Start getting ready for your holistic health care...fill in your own charts for each of the four categories above.

- -

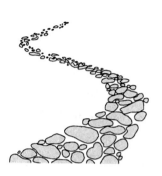

CHAPTER 12
If You Have a Chronic or Serious Issue

The first thing you need to do is drop the idea that your medical insurance needs to cover everything, because they won't...they do not recognize holistic care yet. To take control of your health and get to the other side of your chronic issue, you will have to let go of thinking you can only do what your medical insurance approves of and pays for. They are stuck in their own entrapment of beliefs and cannot help you decide what is best for you.

Second, accept that you have some decisions to make and do not allow ANY doctor, practitioner, or family member to make them for you. Your health care decisions are yours and yours alone to make. That does NOT mean you don't listen to anyone, but instead listen to all opinions and understand that they are coming from the education and experience of the giver. Keep what resonates with you and set aside what doesn't. Repeat this, looking at it all again (even what you have set aside) until you feel confident you have the right answers that fit you.

With our current health care system, doctors barely have time to say hello, let alone meet with other practitioners to discuss your needs. So, as yet anyway, it is up to you to put together all the information you can from the different sources and make your own informed decisions. Let me give you an example. John has operable cancer. The doctor recommends surgery right away, followed by radiation. The holistic care practitioners have shown John there may be other avenues to explore through proper holistic therapies and life style changes.

So, John is faced with two seemingly opposing viewpoints. He needs to be asking questions: "How aggressive is the cancer? How fast is it growing? Am I in immediate danger? How will I know when/if I will be in immediate danger? Can I make the life style changes? Can I really face and deal with my emotional issues? Am I disciplined enough to follow the holistic care routines and diet changes? What are the dangers and side effects for the surgery and radiation, and likewise, for holistic care? When should I be able to see if the holistic route is working? If I choose one will the other still work with me? If I choose both, will the practitioners work together?" Honest answers to these and many more questions will start to reveal to John the best route for him to take.

Step 1: Find your practitioner team.

Pick at least one person from each category, plus your allopathic primary care physician(PC). If you can, choose an IFM/MD or a DO because they already accept holistic care practices. Hopefully, you will be able to find a practitioner or two that can cover more than one category, but if not, that's fine. Definitely include your primary care as well, because they have diagnostic and testing availability that you will not find in energetic care.

Do this BEFORE you need it…it's much easier when you are not in crisis.

- Ask them if they can provide the part of your care you want them to and make it clear where they fit into the overall picture and team. For example: Practitioner A may be able to provide energy balancing and emotional work (say, via five element acupuncture), while Practitioner B can provide mechanical balancing and emotional work (say, via massage and EFT). Choose whether it will be Practitioner A or B who will do the emotional work, and let them both know your decision.

- Make sure they will work well and communicate with the rest of your team and those you have chosen to help.
- Ask what their record keeping is like. Will they be able to get back to and compare their findings from year to year?
- You are hiring them for their expertise and experience that you do not have, but all decisions are yours and yours alone to make.
- Test them out, and keep looking until you find the modalities and practitioners you are comfortable with. For holistic care your personalities need to blend amicably.

Holistic care shines brightest when it comes to prevention. I suggest, at the least, a checkup every other year to catch any changes before they become problems. Use these "checkups" to "check out" your potential practitioners.

Step 2: Make your list of issues, and put them in each of the four categories (physical, emotional, energetic, and nutritional)

Use Chapter 11 for help. If you are in a physical body and live on earth you have issues. (If you really don't think you do, then start your list with denial.) Holistic care practitioners need all the details so we can fit the pieces of the puzzle together, so do not leave anything out. This is unlike allopathic practitioners who do not need to know about anything other than what they are dealing with. Holistic means "all," and we deal with the whole body, mind, and spirit all at once. Every hint helps so we do not think you are a hypochondriac when you give us the details.

Step 3: Make a to-do list in check list form

Make three lists for each of the four stressors: "Do Now," "Need to Accomplish," and "Done." As the Do-Now shortens (moves to Done), move tasks from the Need-To list over to it. This helps in the feeling of accomplishment when the going gets tough.

Step 4: Line up help

Everyone needs support when going through a tough time—that someone who can put things back in perspective, or take over some mundane tasks to give you a break. Of course, this all depends on how serious of an issue you are going through, but, if you have a tough one, get some tough help. If you are experiencing cancer, you may want several people to play different roles, while a minor issue may only require an occasional phone call to a friend.

Remember all those people who said, "Let me know if I can help." Call them! And, give them this book, so they can understand what you want to accomplish. People want to help but they generally don't know how. They want to be helpful, but they don't want to interfere. Talk to them! Give them guidance as to how to deal with this...and with you. If you have a tough issue, you may lose your cool occasionally. Writing down your heart-felt feelings in advance will help your caretaker to continue supporting you even if you said something you regret. Create key words or gestures that will get across what you need in an instant. Then tell them to make their own list for what you need to know about them. Examples:

- Palm facing them = "I can't take this in right now, please do this at another time. I do want to hear it, just not now"

- "Baloney!" = "I'm so frustrated right now, please just let me vent and don't take any of it personally...be my wall!"
- The okay symbol on your heart = "I love you, and I'm sorry, but I have to make this all about me now. Help me get better and I'll make sure it is all about you as soon as I can."

Give each a task. When they don't know what to do for you, tell them the different things you need, and ask which is doable for them. You don't want to overburden your favorite go-to person, so ask and negotiate what they can and are joyfully willing to do. Examples of tasks:

- Researcher – provide a concise written description of modalities, practitioners, side-effects of medications, etc.
- Organizer – keep track of the four categories and their to-do/pending/done lists.
- Scheduler – make or cancel appointments, keep your calendar updated, and assist with keeping you on-course with all four categories.
- Homework scheduler – like Jessie said, remembering the homework can be overwhelming when you don't feel well. A friend can help you make a schedule that you feel good about and keep a daily schedule and log.
- Recap Interloper – This is the friend that you don't see as often, but is good at organizing. They can pull together all that you've accomplished since they saw you last and summarize where you are now (either giving you your comeuppance or showering you with praise...tactfully and lovingly, of course).
- Cook – food prep, recipes or grocery shopping to help you change your diet. This can also be someone who organizes a group of people to provide daily meals if necessary.

- Cheer Leader – Watch a ball game with them, play a game, make jokes and take your mind off the problem for awhile.
- Driver –for appointments and as a second set of ears and note taker.
- Errand Runner – and miscellaneous jobs around the house.
- The Wall – the person you can talk to about anything; bounce ideas off; and help you see through yourself to the answers. Note: this is not the bossy person who wants to make the decisions for you. This is the one who helps YOU make the decisions.

On your better days, make sure you let them know you appreciate what they are doing for you. And remember, if you are having a hard time with it, it's okay to make it all about you. Helping others and being helped is about keeping the exchange of energy even. If it's your turn to receive, take it graciously. When it's their turn, give it, equally as graciously. (You may want to reread the section *Owning Your Own Power* in Chapter 6.)

Step 5: Accept the task of "getting there"

It took you a long time to create a chronic issue, so accept that it may take a while to fix it. Accept that, and strap yourself in for the ride.

Remain unattached to the outcome. Find the trust that you will be able to become the best that you can be with what you have. You may, or may not, be able to totally fix the issue, but you WILL be able to improve your life. HOW it improves is what you need to remain flexible and unattached about.

If you are resisting and still just want it to go away without doing the work, you may want to start with some emotional work that will help you accept the task. You never know—bringing yourself into alignment may be your key to your house of cards.

Step 6: Get to work

Stay organized in your mind: What stage are you in? Getting started? The grind? The roller coaster? Don't give up? Redoing the plan? If you're in the middle of a tough issue, you will most likely be going back and forth through these stages...they are not linear. Knowing where you are; why it is happening; and that it's normal, can do wonders for speeding up and easing your ride.

What issues are coming up? Keep the lists going and updated. Things come up for release in layers, so you may need to revisit parts of the list that had already moved to "done". It can be frustrating to have to visit the same issue again, but know it is just another layer and accept it—accept that it's frustrating, and keep going.

Step 7: Stay focused on your intent

It's easy to focus on what you are going through instead of where you are going, so make the effort to keep imagining the desired result. Again, all those people that said they would like to help— put them to work imagining what fun things they will be doing with you when you are well again.

Step 8: Rejoice in the accomplishments

The roller coaster ride feels like many setbacks, but for each of those there will be more leaps ahead. Rejoice in them. Have something you do with your helper team that celebrates them. It will raise your frequency because it is happy. It will re-affirm the positive thinking and help your subconscious learn your new ways.

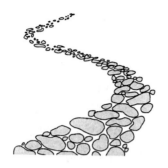

CHAPTER 13
If You Are Helping Someone Else

Know your role as their friend and what it is you are willing and able to provide. It's open communication, always. Re-read Chapter 12 so you know what their perspective may be. Buy them their own copy of this book, but don't force your ideas on them. If they are drawn to it, great. If not, it may not be their path.

If you're unsure of what they want from you, ask. If they are unclear, offer to do the tasks you know you can do comfortably. If you're afraid to have this open communication, look at your own stuff and do your Whys and Yea-buts so you can speak your mind with tact and compassion. They may be the one going through "getting there", but you will be learning about yourself, too.

Ask questions, instead of making statements, and give ideas to think about, instead of opinions about how they should think. It's hard enough being sick and needing help, so the last thing that's needed is someone telling you what to do and making you feel even more incapable. So instead of saying, "You should...," ask, "Have you thought about ...?" Then listen.

Ask them to make a list of words and gestures that give you clues as to what they want. They will be able to use them in an instant without effort or concern that you will take their words the wrong way.

Make a list of words and gestures that indicate what you mean when the words are hard to say. Plan in advance how you might handle the tough things if they happen. This helps your conscious mind take control so you don't get sucked into their drama...so you can handle it tactfully and keep your stress level even. Some examples:

- "I need to be heard, can you do that now?"
- "I love you, but I need a break."
- "I'm so sorry, but I can't provide that right now...how else can I help?"
- "I can't rearrange that part of my schedule. Can I call someone who may be able to do it then?

Know that it's all about them right now. If the energy is uneven and you become reluctant to continue, investigate why that is (do your own Whys and Yea-buts) to get back on an even keel. They may be taking advantage of you or not appreciating what you do. Or, you may not be speaking up about your needs and thus giving too much of yourself away. Or you may be afraid of letting them down if your circumstances have changed and you cannot provide as much. Any of these scenarios requires you to look at your stuff, and take action to even out the energy imbalances. Even though they are the ones in need right now, it's okay to take care of yourself first. Otherwise, there will be nothing left in you to give.

Do not be the enabler. As an example, if they are taking advantage, that is very likely one of the lessons they need to learn to get over their illness. Do not deny them their learning experience by hiding your feelings from them...it serves no one. Be tactful, kind, and empathetic. Appraise which are your issues and which are theirs. Fix your own stuff, and speak your truth. If they react poorly to your feelings, know it is theirs to deal with and it's your job to bring on the compassion without getting dragged into their stuff.

Let them take their own path. If you have knowledge that they do not possess, it is your task to share it with them. It is NOT your task to judge whether they use the information or not. This is their life, and no one else knows what their purpose is. So, as mentioned before, judging what is best for someone else is arrogance. However, that being said, there are circumstances where a more forceful "taking control" is warranted. For example: they may be too depleted to care enough to make the hard choice; or they may have severe issues about receiving, so automatically tell you no. Be VERY careful with this. Check your ego, talk it over with others who have different perspectives, and make sure you are doing what the person you are in charge of really wants. They will give you signs along the way, so pay attention.

Know their schedule, who the other helpers are (if any), what their jobs are and work cooperatively with everyone. Read chapter 12, so you can help them do a better job of communicating their needs.

Do not take what they are going through personally. Catch yourself when you are simply reacting and stop the emotional train ride by separating yourself from the event. (✍ Be the Observer) They may be feeling down, but they don't want you to be down, too. Find your balance between sympathy and getting sucked into their mood. Sometimes they will really want your opinion. Sometimes they'll want you to agree with them. Sometimes they will want you to be their sounding board so they can hear what they are saying through different words. And sometimes, they will just want to vent and know there will be no judgment.

Most importantly, be yourself. You are friends with this person because of who you are, and, it can happen, but it's usually not the time to be changing your role in the relationship. Allow any changes to evolve and grow naturally. For example, if you have always been the guy that made jokes and went to football games with your friend, you will probably be better off signing up for the task of "cheerleader" rather than "organizer."

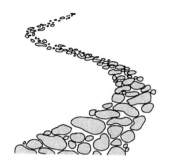

CHAPTER 14

If You Are a Holistic Practitioner

Resolve your own anger about our current health care system. During this time of change and chaos, establishing yourself as a legitimate holistic care practitioner can be difficult. Make sure you resolve any anger and frustration about allopathic medicine, pharmaceutical companies, and medical insurance companies. As you know, holding these emotions will lower your frequency and therefore, your ability to help your client. It may help to read the next two chapters slowly.

Manage expectations. The hard part about holistic care is you often do not know just what it was that worked for a particular client. Following are three examples of why it is so important to educate your clients, as well as the general public whenever possible. Managing expectations is a big part of the job.

1) No "one" thing: Here in the USA, we've grown up with, "you take this pill and it fixes that problem"—there is a one to one relationship, and what you did to fix something is most often known. For chronic issues many things need to be addressed, and there usually is no "one" thing that finally topples the house of cards. In holistic care it's up to

the practitioners to help their clients' expectations of knowing exactly what worked. We are all different and there are infinite ways their issue could have been created, so there are also infinite ways to resolve it.

2) Clients may never know: Since holistic care is still so new to so many, it presents another problem for the practitioners—clients may never know what you did was a big part in their healing, simply because they don't understand what you did. My clients often had significant improvement in one or two sessions, but could not relate that the sessions may have had something to do with it. This is a nice-to-have problem because you are helping people, but it does nothing for your marketing. Education IS your marketing.

3) Wanting the miracle: Some clients are the opposite: wanting the miracle and holding out hope that you are it. It can be tricky to help clients understand that there is no magic answer and at the same time help them to think positively that they can improve.

Learn some of the body signs. You don't need to know a lot about them (unless that's your specialty of course), but if you're a body worker, you can do your clients a great service if you can tell them when an indicator has changed. You can start by being familiar with the Body Babble list in Appendix A, or by learning a few key acupressure points. Have a list of practitioners that you work well with for each of the four categories, so you can refer clients out when you find something that needs further investigation. Your clients will love you for keeping an eye on things and helping them to find issues early.

Know your clients expectations of you and whether you can provide it or not, then work towards that end. Some want their chief complaint dealt with first and don't understand that some other things may have to be fixed before you can get to it. Make sure they know you ARE dealing with the complaint they came to you for.

Be confident, be humble, know your scope of practice: always make sure you are grounded, and stay neutral to what happens.

Continue to work on your own stuff. We are all continuously growing and changing. If you are in the business of caring for others, you need to take good care of yourself, and this includes continuous work on your own issues. Your client base will sometimes point you in the right direction. For example, say you have an unusual number of clients with shoulder issues. Because likes attract, it could be a signal to take a look at yourself. Are you physically overworking your shoulder? Are you beginning to feel overwhelmed (like you have the weight of the world on your shoulders)? Practice what you preach and investigate yourself.

Don't take yourself so seriously. Make a mistake? We all do. Admit it and learn from it so it doesn't happen again…then move on. Analyzing it to death or carrying guilt about it, does not serve you or your client. If you've read this far, you've heard about a few of mine!

Truth…what is that really? We can speak our own truth, but when it comes to clients and our intuitive hits about them, it may feel like truth to us, but is it their Truth with a capital T? Is it the truth for the moment? For a particular situation? For this reality or another? Only when the client resonates with it and claims it as theirs does it become "Truth" that you can move forward with. Be careful of assumptions. For the practitioner, intuitive hits are information that belongs to the client, and it's our job to give it to them to interpret. We can assist them in the process by giving them ideas or suggestions, but it is their reaction to those ideas that label it as truth, Truth, or false.

Accept that you may never know why? As mentioned above, with holistic care the client works with many aspects at the same time, so they (nor you) may never know what actually did the trick...it's all of it, it's all related.

Introduce yourself to the allopathic medical community so they know who you are, what you do, and how you can help their patients. Help the doctors get to know you by offering a discount to the first few patients they send to you. Be a team player. Respect what they do, and they will more likely respect what you do. It's cooperation that is building the new holistic care system.

Stop fighting regulation. Holistic care has been on the outside looking in when it comes to regulation. We've seen what it's doing to our medical system—how it shackles the doctors from doing their best—and we don't want any part of it. In our world, regulation has become synonymous with "unfair." Our clients have very few indicators of who are legitimate practitioners and who are the charlatans, so we have to acknowledge that some additional regulation and licensing is necessary. It won't do us any good to bury our heads in the sand, so I suggest we start talking about it...get some great ideas together and get them out there in the energy to manifest in a totally new way that benefits both clients and practitioners.

Build your own team: whether it is all in one office or a group that works well together. If not you, know who can provide quality care for the four stress groups.

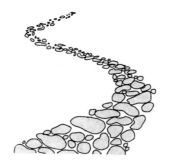

CHAPTER 15
If You Are an Allopathic Doctor

We are in the middle of massive changes and this can be quite frustrating to all those involved. (Note: You may want to re-read the section, *Why Holistic Health Care Is So Hard.*)

I, for one, very much appreciate those of you who are already making the transition to thinking more holistically. Thank you... the world needs you.

For those who have not yet, I understand the difficulty in switching a lifetime of beliefs and career building to something brand new. Usually this is done through attrition—those that believe the old ways slowly phase out to be replaced by new thinking generations. This process is started by a few brave souls who dare to be different—who can withstand the ridicule; being ostracized; and being called quacks by their peers. If the new thinking has merit, then eventually they are joined by more brave souls. Then scientists and accepted organizations join in to prove them either right or wrong. If proven right, educational systems start teaching the new way...and this grows until only a few of those believing the old ways are left. They become the ones being ridiculed; ostracized; and called "has-beens"...until they, too, retire and leave it to the younger generations. Normally this is a long transition that takes four or more generations to complete.

This is the cycle we are currently in (after the science community has proven it right, and some MDs have already moved to the new way of thinking). The problem is the need for change is so great, that the transition is happening in about half the time. This means the "old guard" is (and will be) forced to change before they are ready. This, can be very difficult. For those of you not in this position, imagine building your education and career around models that you believe help people, only to find out later in life that some of these models are wrong. This can be a devastating jolt to one's nervous system and psyche. This is what is being asked of our established MDs. In terms of history, it is happening very fast, but it cannot happen overnight for an individual.

It helps to know that generally, holistic care practitioners are NOT in opposition to MDs, but we do work in opposite fundamentals. We work "with" the body to help it heal itself, while you do things "to" the body. We are more about prevention, while you are more about fixing what is already wrong. We need them both! Yes, you are the ones with the degrees that the law will side with and we genuinely want to work with you! However, you also must respect our skills and understand that when it comes to energy, digestion, essential oils, herbs, spirituality, and the emotions associated with pain and illness, we know more than you do— that's where we have been trained and you have not. We do not know about pharmaceuticals, surgery, diagnostic machines, blood test, etc.—that is where you are trained and we are not. Again, we specialize in prevention; you in fixing what's already symptomatic. You already refer to other specialists for their specific expertise...just do the same with holistic practitioners, even though you don't totally understand it...you don't need to. Simply understand the fundamental difference, and use it to your patient's advantage. Just for a minute, imagine the medical system we can create if we work together.

There are already organizations in place that can help you make the transitions, but instead, they are working against you— by taking away your freedom to truly help; by squeezing your time to unbelievably short; and by restricting payments so it becomes impossible to do the job you originally wanted to do. And worse, they have locked you into the hamster wheel, so you have neither the time nor the ambition to right this system.

This is not because the organizations are inherently evil and intentionally doing this (well maybe some are, but most are not, so we're not going there). When things come about so gradually, like the evolution of our health care system, it becomes increasingly hard to see the flaws within it because we are so immersed and have known it for so long. This makes it difficult to even think about another way. From that, the flaws are built upon the flaws, until finally it is way out of the strike zone of usefulness. It is so large and imbedded in society, that it will take a complete collapse or revolution to change it. We are in the middle of that revolution. I am asking you to be a part of it, so we can make it through this massive change without the collapse and make sure the revolution is resolution from which we can build better and better.

So, Doctor, the change is happening whether you are a part of it or not. Most likely there will be plenty of people who still believe in the allopathic ways to keep those of you busy until you retire, but I am hoping you will be one of the brave souls who help make the change instead of letting the change happen TO you.

Science continues to evolve, and many of the things we thought years ago to be true have been proven false. And, there will be many things that are proven true today that will be proven false in years to come. This is an eternal process as we forever expand our knowledge, so it is up to all of us to be flexible in our beliefs and evolve along with the endlessly expanding knowledge.

What can Doctors do?

- Accept that there are new and valid methods of healthcare.
- Accept that you have a part to play in fixing what is wrong with the current system.
- Investigate osteopathic medicine and functional medicine to see if they are a direction you'd like to go.[14]
- Consider building a team of your own (either within your practice or along with other practices where you work together) that will cover the "other" three stressors (energy, emotions, digestion)
- Devote an hour a week to learning something new about holistic care; how you can help fix what is wrong; or imagining how you would like your practice to be (setting your intent). You can start by getting familiar with the ideas in this book.
- Make a goal of introducing yourself to the holistic care practitioners near you... three per year as an example. Negotiate a rigorously discounted rate for the first few patients you send there so you can establish trust in their work and their communication methods.
- Keep pushing back the restrictions from the institutions by writing letters; calling your legislators; speaking up at conferences; and encouraging your medical universities to catch up to the new sciences and discoveries.

- Talk to your colleagues…we all like company in the way we think. The more doctors who cooperate with holistic care and talk about it, the more comfortable it becomes for everyone, and the sooner we can all work out the kinks.
- Create the energy of what you want by using your imagination. For example: imagine what it will be like when we all work together—you have more time to truly help people with what you know; costs are under control; you are paid well; and you are part of a team that is building the best health care system the world has ever seen.

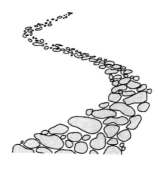

CHAPTER 16

If You Are in Medical Insurance, Education, or Regulation

Okay, let's get real here. The current business of medical insurance is not sustainable…this is business planning 101, and it seems like those actually in the business (along with our legislatures) are the only ones who can't see that.

Our medical system model is changing (which is what this book is all about). That means those in the medical insurance business have to change also or it's belly up for you. Harsh tones? Yes, but someone needs to wake people up who play in this industry.

Let's go back to the basics…insurance is supposed to be about spreading the cost of a catastrophe over a large number of people and over time. People are willing to pay into this over time to make sure (INsure) they will not be hit with large costs all at once, if something does happen. These payments given to the insurance companies cover their costs of operations; pay the employees; provide reasonable profits so they can continue to improve their company; and build funds to pay out when a catastrophe actually does happen.

Simple? Yes. But here's the problem: That is not what the medical insurance in the USA is doing. They are expected to pay for all health care costs AND cover the catastrophic occurrences. This takes them out of the realm of simple insurance and puts them squarely in the middle of payment broker for all health care costs. This is what gives them unprecedented control of our health care, simply by establishing what they will and will not pay for. We, John Q. Public, over time have sat back and allowed this to happen. How? We let them control what we do by dutifully following what they tell us to do through what they will pay for. Our country has fallen into some very destructive habits in our thinking:

- "If my insurance doesn't cover it, it must not be any good"
- "I am paying all this money every month, so I am not going to pay out of pocket too, even if it is a better solution."
- "Our medical system and my doctor know what they are doing, so who am I to question what they suggest?"
- "The medical system is responsible for my health...I can do and eat whatever I want, and they will fix it...that's what I'm paying for.

In order for this model to work even slightly well, people have to be treated all the same. There have to be rules set up to "diagnose" and "treat" exactly the same way every time. There is no wiggle room for anyone who does not fit the mold, and patients and doctors alike feel this as entrapment. Consequently, this is how our medical system has been built...it has to match the insurance model of "everyone is diagnosed and treated the same way."

But, something new is happening out here in John Q. Public's world. We are discovering that this model has forbidden new ideas and ways of thinking...that this model does not work for most people because we are all NOT the same. The doctors working within it are frustrated about being stuck in the rules of payment instead of doing what is best for the patient. So, guess what? Many of them are leaving the insurance-based system and starting their practices based on private pay. And guess what? Those that can afford their own costs are dumping their insurance plans and taking responsibility for their own health and associated costs. What does this eventually do? More and more healthy people are leaving the system, leaving the majority that is left in the less healthy category, (which have higher costs and less income to pay). For the insurance companies this is clearly not sustainable. As more and more people seek what really works for them, the current insurance models will soon be out of business altogether, leaving the only answer an entirely tax funded arm of the government.

Jessie's story is a typical example of the financial advantage of including holistic care in what insurance covers and treating patients as individuals. The cost savings of the drugs she is no longer taking would pay for her eight months of holistic care in only a couple of years. And, that is not counting the savings from fewer doctor visits and tests or any future increases in drugs that may have been needed. Plus, she now has the tools and knowledge to continue decreasing her health care costs. Holistic care IS economical, and, in my opinion, the only way to dig ourselves out of the staggering costs of our allopathic system.

Here is an example of "cost control" controlling care, but not actually controlling costs. I went to the doctor for a check up which included blood tests. She asked me if I had insurance. When I replied, "No", she said, "Oh, good. That means I can get you the better blood tests. They actually cost less too, but the insurance companies won't cover them." (Really? This is insane.)

For a long time, we all bought into "we are not responsible for ourselves." We expected our doctors to know everything, and fix whatever we did to ourselves with a simple pill. We made them responsible for us, and they took it on by becoming the boss of our health and we followed everything they said without question or thought. (Talk about two sides of the same coin feeding each other...egads...look what we created!)

Which came first? You can see the pattern clearly in this example (with "we" as John Q. Public and "they" as the doctors):

- We told them they were responsible for us by suing them whenever something went wrong;
- Their costs for liability insurance skyrocketed;
- We created the attitude of, "I don't have to worry about taking care of myself—that's the doctor's job";
- They developed "cover their asses" attitudes and methods of practice such as extra tests and duplications;
- That in turn raised costs;
- Everyone began to think, "Don't worry about the costs, the medical insurance will pay";
- So the insurance companies became more about controlling costs than helping people.
- In the mean time, no one was paying attention to the deeply ingrained system we were really building.
- Now, it is so ingrained in all aspects of our system that it's a massive effort to turn it around.

So what can be done?

Be a participant!

- If you are in medical insurance, recognize that it has to change or you may all be out of jobs sooner than you want. Start talking about it with colleagues. Change the energy around your desk with affirmations and imagining the solutions. That will help others to start doing the same thing…it's a ground up effort, not top down.

- If you are in medical education, start suggesting that holistic classes should be offered along with history about how our medical system became as it is (still so young compared to others). Teach how to build a holistic care practice. Come up with ideas of how to change the residency and internship training to better fit today's world instead of perpetuating what has always been.

- If you are in regulation, take a good hard look at the laws protecting this old and failing system, and come up with ways to support the new. Start by publicly recognizing that holistic care modalities are real and legitimate. Support those small businesses working in that arena. Understand that the current system will soon collapse if changes are not made.

Will it be the insurance companies that create themselves anew? Which one of you will be the visionary to restructure your company so it can survive by stepping out of the "payment and cost control" model and stepping back into a "spread the cost of catastrophe" model?

Will it be government that wakes up and forces the ship to turn around with new laws and regulations? Are any of you brave enough to go against the establishment of legislatures, lobbyists, and PACS with some new ideas of your own?

Will it be the schools that finally start teaching what is needed instead of what has always been?

Those that step up will be the winners and those that don't will be left in their dust. Which one will you be? This holistic train cannot be stopped, because it has reached the speed of no return.

Enough people have awakened that we long ago reached the hundredth monkey of mass consciousness for this change.

"Polly-Anna," you say? "You don't know what you're talking about," you say? Take a look around you, there is change in the direction I speak of everywhere. Does it really make sense to have our medical treatments controlled by those with no medical background? I am stating the obvious to those who are not blinded by the old ways.

Come on everyone! I know we can do better. Walk out of the forest so you can see what is really happening, and then we can catch this collapse before it happens and create a truly great and affordable health care system that moves from a model of what NOT to do, to a model the rest of the world will want to emulate.

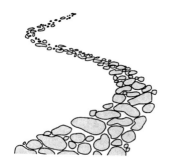

EPILOGUE

"Getting there" is a multilayered process. The first "there" may start with the desire to get over a chronic illness or pain, but when that is completed another "there" is defined, and then another, and another. You've learned how to navigate holistic care from wherever you are to wherever you want to be. And I hope you've learned that getting to wellness is only the beginning. The same methods are used to get to abundance, happiness, accomplishments, relationships, balance, and the sheer joy for life.

I invite you to exploit this book by using it as your journal to "there"...write in it; refer to it; add your story to it; and compare last year's answers to the Challenges and Body Babble to this year's. Let this book get dog-eared and worn.

If you walk away from reading this book with only one thing, let it be this: What we label as "bad times" are only our challenges that push us to become better; to find our power; and to be more mindful creators. Switching our thinking from identifying events as "bad times" to believing they are "another adventure" will carry you farther than any other advice I can give.

Life is for living and experiencing it all—the good, the bad, the ugly, and the beautiful, because it is ALL part of the natural balancing of energy. It is ALL fragments of the unconditional love symphony that has been separated out for the purpose of experiencing all of its parts. This is how we learn about love and our creative power. This is how we learn to make life happen instead of letting it happen to us. This is how we, not only get well, but become great.

So enjoy all of the parts of this journey we call life. We are all on it together…learning, teaching, growing, and receiving. Find the laughter in the mistakes; the smiles after the anger; and the forgiveness after the hurt. The world becomes more beautiful with each triumph; more expanded with each challenge; and more awesome with each little awakening. See beyond it all, as the world always balancing itself, pulling itself and us with it back to equilibrium. Don't sweat the small stuff, but LIVE it…it all has a purpose.

You have a purpose.

Notes for Year _____

Notes for Year _____

Notes for Year _____

Notes for Year _____

Notes for Year _____

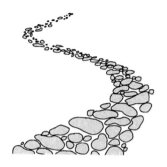

Appendix A

"Anything inside is bound to manifest outwardly.
Outward manifestations and their locality may reveal
the conditions of the internal organs;
in this way, the location of the illness will be known."

"Treatise on the Original Organs" *in Miraculous Pivot*

—Liu Yanchi—

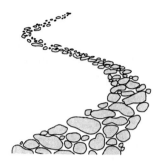

Body Babble

This section is all about "**HINTS**." The best way to use it is to write down (every year) each ping you have and compare the result to prior years. Then let the changes you see in the lists be a guide as you work with your professionals to figure out what they mean.

NOTE: This list is **NOT MY EXPERTISE**, but it is my accumulated information from my many years of study. It is **NOT COMPLETE**, so I encourage you to write in this book the additional Body Babble signs you run across in your journey. I will also add more to the list on my website as I learn them.

Please read!!

These Body Babble signs are **NOT A DIAGNOSIS**, but **THEY ARE HINTS** about what MAY be in your future if you don't pay attention. Each sign by itself tells you nothing. Many things need to be taken into consideration: Were you born with it; has it changed; does it come and go; did a past injury cause it; and are there other signs that indicate the same thing? The body does not just give you one hint if something is amiss...it will give you several. Take them as a guide as to what you can investigate to find out more.

Again, I do not want you getting all nervous if you have several of these Body Babble signs. Remember, your body is guiding you, and it lets you know way ahead of time if something may go wrong in your future. This list is about listening to the whispers and taking action to PREVENT your body yelling at you later with illnesses and pain.

Here is some additional information to help you understand this list:

- Yeast goes hand-in-hand with not enough pro-biotics, because with any pro-biotic, if there is not enough of one, then another may be able to overgrow and vise-versa. That is why I recommend taking different brands of probiotics to make sure you get a good balance. For example, when you finish a bottle, the next one should have a different composition. (See point 3 in *More about Nutrition*, Chapter 3)
- Not enough proteins, carbs, or fats can be because of diet, not breaking them down, or not absorbing them.
- "Check Digestion" means take each of the four functions into account: what you take in, its breakdown, absorbing it, and eliminating it.
- The thyroid uses iodine, so anything that indicates an iodine deficiency hints at thyroid stress, and vice-versa.
- Most of the hints are about deficiency unless otherwise indicated as an "excess" hint, but when investigating, always consider both excess and deficiency.
- Some vitamins and minerals need to be accompanied by protein or fat because they "ride" on them in order to get to the cells. Magnesium, for example needs protein, so it's better taken with a meal that contains protein.

- Sodium can show as deficient if your intake of it is mostly the "white" salt (processed) and not the natural salts, such as sea salt or Himalayan salt.

General Body

- Roving aches/pains = not enough calcium
- Aneurysms = not enough copper or vitamin C
- Spider veins = not enough copper or vitamin C
- Chemical sensitivity = too much yeast (Candida)
- Feel cold often = not enough iodine, or weak thyroid, look at calcium and vitamin D also.
- PH usually low (acidic) = not digesting proteins, too much sugar in diet
- Edema (swelling or retaining water) = leaky gut where proteins or carbs are escaping into the blood.
- Fissures or hemorrhoids = check vitamin C, yeast, and probiotics
- Growth issues or petite stature = lack of protein or magnesium, check pituitary
- Weak immune system = the immune system needs protein, vitamin A, C, D, zinc, and selenium. Also check for low grade infection, such as lymes disease, or teeth.
- Food sensitivities = need for enzymes , weak immune system, or sensitive to GMOs (genetically modified organisms), pesticides or fertilizers
- Mucus membranes inflamed, red, itchy = check sodium levels
- Odor that is different = check zinc
- Premature aging = too much yeast
- Shaky or tremors = check fat intake and digestion, too much yeast.
- Thirsty, not relieved by drinking water = not enough trace minerals

- Excess water secretions (watery eyes, excess spit, etc) = not digesting proteins and leaky gut
- Do not tolerate exercise = protein deficiencies
- Weakness general = check water intake and copper, gluten sensitivity
  - Not enough Endurance = check iodine
  - Energy lacking = check vitamin B, E and digestion of carbs
  - Fatigue = check carbs, water, potassium, selenium, sodium and vitamin B
  - Fatigue mid-afternoon = check iodine as well
  - Tired = check vitamin C
- Weight Issues = not digesting proteins or carbs or too much yeast
  - Barrel chested = pay close attention to lungs
  - Firm weight all over = pay close attention to heart and insulin levels
  - Pear shape = pay close attention to liver and hormone levels
  - Soft squishy weight all over = pay close attention to your spleen

Abdomen

- Bloating / gas / indigestion = maybe need enzymes, probiotics, or overabundance of yeast
- Firm beer belly = check vitamin C, B-5
- Flabby Belly = check thyroid and iodine
- Heartburn / gerd = are you chest breathing? May need enzymes or more water. Use of antacids can cause lack of protein
- Frequent nausea = are you drinking enough water, kidney stress
  - With poor appetite = too much vitamin D

- Constipation = not digesting carbs
- Diarrhea = not digesting proteins

Arms/legs

- Knee/elbow has crusty skin = possible hypothyroid
- Muscle cramps = check water intake, possible lack of magnesium (see Muscles)
- Joint pain = see Bones
- Tenderness on inside of leg at and just below knee = toxicity overload

Back

- Disc problems = not enough protein or not digesting it
- Spinal pain (neck, back, low back) = check water intake, no artificial sweeteners, maybe too much sugar
- Poor posture = check calcium
- Protrusion between C6, C7 at base of neck = check iodine
- Thickening between shoulder blades = check iodine

Blood

- Anemia = check copper, iron, vitamin B-9 and B-12
- Excess bleeding = check iodine, vitamin C
- Slow clotting time = check calcium
- Too thick or too thin = not digesting fats, if too thick check water intake
- History of clots or strokes = check vitamin E
- Diagnosed low oxygen levels = check iodine and iron, not digesting fats
- Pale color to either skin or blood =check iron
- High LDL cholesterol = check magnesium

- Low HDL cholesterol = check chromium
- High blood pressure = not digesting proteins or fats, not enough water, check magnesium, potassium, selenium, and sodium
- Bl. pressure up/down (not controlled) = not digesting fats
- Sugar imbalances = can produce too much yeast (it feeds on sugar)
  - Diabetes II, hypoglycemia, high triglycerides = check chromium, iron, sugar and carb intake
  - Low blood sugar = check sodium
  - If cause is enzyme imbalance = check manganese
- Low white blood cell count = check copper, vitamin A

Bones

- Brittle, or osteoporosis, or thinning = check vitamin D, manganese, magnesium, calcium
- Joint pain = check water intake, possible excess iron, too much sugar, GMO sensitivity, eliminate artificial sweeteners
- Stiffness = check sodium and water intake
- TMJ, clicking in jaw = not digesting proteins

Breasts

- Fibrocystic = check iodine and thyroid
- Fluid retention = check vitamin E
- Tenderness = check vitamin E

Diseases

- Auto-immune diseases (any) = check vitamin D, gluten sensitivity
- Bells Palsy = check calcium, magnesium, vitamin B
- Carpel tunnel = check vitamin B-6

- Fainting or dizzy when rising = check vitamin B-6
- Genetic = check vitamin A
- Morning sickness = check vitamin B-6
- Motion sickness = check vitamin B-6
- Rickets = vitamin D
- Syndrome X (HPB, high triglycerides, Blood sugar issues, low HDL, hrt disease) = check chromium
- Diagnosed pancreas issues = check calcium, magnesium, potassium, add enzymes to meals

Ears

- Ringing or hearing loss = check vitamin D
- An angled crease in ear lobe = keep an eye on heart and circulation
- Clicking in ears when moving jaw = not digesting proteins

Endocrine system (hormones)

- Adrenal Issues = not digesting proteins or fats, check sodium, vitamin C, B-5, yeast overload, caffeine and sugar intake
- Difficulty regulating hormones = not digesting proteins or fats, NSAIDS can cause hormone deficiency,
- T3 low on blood tests (thyroid) = check selenium

Eyes

- Blood shot eyes = check vitamin B-2
- Circles under the eyes
  - More towards nose = check adrenals, vitamin C, B-5,
  - More towards outer edge = check kidneys
  - Inside corner above the eye = check spleen
  - Red = allergies to something, not digesting carbs

- Trouble focusing when distance changes = check zinc
- Dry, burning, or puffy = not digesting carbs, too much yeast
- Floaters = check sodium, spleen, lymphatic system, toxin levels
- Glaucoma = check chromium
- Eye lashes angle towards nose = check PH for too acidic, for diet reduce carbs and meat, increase leafy greens
- Macular degeneration = not digesting proteins, may need lutein, antioxidants
- Near sightedness = check vitamin D
- Poor night vision = check vitamin A
- Excess tears, or watery by lashes = not digesting proteins, check vitamin B-2
- Pupil enlarged or pulsing = check adrenals, sugar and caffeine intake
- Hooded eyelid (skin between eyebrow and lid hangs over lid) = check liver, and toxin intake

Gallbladder

- Removed = check digestion of proteins, lecithin, vitamin A

Hair

- Dry / lusterless = not digesting fats, check vitamin F
- Oily = eating the wrong fats and not digesting them
- Falling out = not digesting fats, check iodine, vitamin B
- Gray prematurely = check copper and trace minerals
- Scaly scalp = yeast overload
- Thinning (loss pattern)
  - Top = check iodine and thyroid (hypothyroid)
  - Temporal region (sides) = check kidneys
  - Front top = check lungs

- Crown = not digesting proteins
- Side burns = check gall bladder
- Both temporal and front top = check toxin overload

Hands and Feet

- Generally cold = not digesting proteins, check iodine
- Nerve issues = check vitamin B
- Smelly feet = check zinc
- Hands turn in when standing relaxed (back of hand facing front) = not digesting proteins, check thyroid
- Tingling or loss of feeling = check vitamin E
- Large toe bent towards next tow = check liver
- Small toe bent inward = check kidney
- Extra long second toe = may have more stomach issues than the norm
- Heal cracks = metal toxicity, possible yeast overload
- Heavy on the heals when walking = check calcium
- Swelling of hands and/or feet = not digesting proteins

Head / Face

- Head aches = check water intake, iron, yeast overload,
- If migraines = also check vitamin B-3
- Eye brow—missing outer third = check iodine and thyroid
- Acne = check chromium, vitamin C, probiotics, and yeast overload
  - Dry/white/thready = check vitamin B
  - On the jaw line = check bowels and elimination part of digestion
  - Slow healing = check zinc
  - White heads = check vitamin B-2
- Cheeks red = check lungs

- Lines in forehead have a broken pattern = check adrenal stress
- Deep wrinkle between brow, center or right = check liver, center or left = check spleen
- Mustache in females = check liver and adrenals
- Zipper lip wrinkles = check hormone imbalance, not digesting fats
- Red in diamond area formed by nose, chin, mouth = check digestion
- TMJ tension = not digesting proteins
- Hardness or lumps under jaw bone = not digesting carbs

Heart

- Irregular beat or palpitations = check potassium, sodium, vitamin B-3
- Rapid beat = check calcium, magnesium
- Blood pressure issues = check calcium, magnesium
- Circulation issues = check vitamin E, B-3,
- Diagnosed oxidation issues = check vitamin E
- Diagnosed heart disease = check copper
  - or vascular disease = check magnesium, vitamin B-9
  - or muscle weakness = magnesium, potassium, sodium, vitamin B-9

Large Intestines

- Colitis or Crohnes = probiotics, yeast overload, reduce carbs and sugars, take enzymes that include cellulase
- Cramps or constipation = not digesting carbs, not enough water, check potassium or an excess of vitamin D
- Gas, bloating, distention of belly = not breaking food down (need enzymes), yeast overload, or need probiotics

- Irritable bowel (IBS) = check magnesium, not breaking food down (need enzymes), yeast overload, or need probiotics

Liver

- Diagnosed issues with bile formation = check magnesium
- Diagnosed liver disease = check for excess iron
- Diagnosed metabolic function problems = check magnesium

Lungs / Respiratory

- Can't take a deep breath = not digesting fats
- Breath with chest instead of abdomen = check vitamin C, PH for acidity,
- Allergies = check probiotics and yeast overgrowth, if child under 5 check histidine (an amino acid)
  - Nightshade vegetable sensitivity = check vitamin B-3
  - Wheat sensitivity = check magnesium
- Asthma = check vitamin E, probiotics, yeast overgrowth
- Impaired breathing = check copper, vitamin B-3

Mental / brain

- Clarity of mind is lacking = check magnesium and zinc
- Hard to concentrate = not digesting carbs
- Dyslexia = check vitamin B-12
- History of brain injury = check digestion of fats
- Insomnia = check calcium, vitamin C, B-5, probiotics, yeast overload, potassium
- Learning disability = check manganese
- Poor memory = yeast overgrowth
- Nervousness = check calcium, sodium, vitamin D
- Restlessness = check overall digestion

- Reading comprehension = check iodine (thyroid)
- ADD, ADHD, OCD = not digesting fats
  - ADD with fatigue = not digesting carbs, check potassium
- Anxiety = check water intake, and digestion (breakdown of foods, may need enzymes supplement)
- Apathy (indifference) = check potassium (especially after giving birth)
- Suppressed appetite = check vitamin B1, B3
- Chronic Fatigue = probiotics, yeast overgrowth, not digesting carbs, potassium
- Confusion = check chromium
- Cravings – general = overall digestion, especially probiotics, excess yeast
  - Alcohol = check potassium
  - Chocolate = check magnesium
  - Salty = check sodium
  - Salty & crunchy = not digesting proteins
  - Sugar = not digesting fats, or carbs
- Difficulty making decisions = not digesting proteins, liver stress
- Depression = not digesting proteins, water intake
  - Suicidal = check iodine (hypothyroid indicated)
- Mental Fatigue = not digesting proteins (hydrochloric acid disruption)
- Dizziness = check sodium, trace minerals, yeast overgrowth
- Eating disorder = check zinc
- Hunger, but for what is unknown = not digesting proteins
- Irritability or anxiousness = check chromium, selenium, water intake
- Mood swings = probiotics, yeast overgrowth
- Not the normal maternal instincts = check manganese, potassium

- MS = not digesting fats
- Hyper or hypo conditions = check magnesium
- Sensitivity to sudden noises (startles) = not digesting carbs, check vitamin B-1
- Can't handle stress = not digesting proteins, check vitamin B-5

Mouth

- Bad breath = yeast overgrowth
  - One hour after eating = not digesting proteins (hydrochloric acid disruption)
- Corners of lips cracked = check vitamin B-12
- Dry = may be due to medications, not digesting carbs
- Inflamed = check iron
- Excess saliva = not digesting proteins
- Sores, or canker sores = check PH for acidity, not digesting carbs or fats
- Loss of taste = check zinc
- Bottom lip bigger than top lip = sign of constipation = not digesting carbs
- Loose teeth or receding gums = not digesting proteins
- Bleeding gums = not digesting proteins, check vitamin C
- Tooth decay = check calcium, vitamin D
- Tongue (stick your tongue out to check)
  - Tip quivers or rounded up = check magnesium, adrenals
  - Scalloped edges (teeth indents remain) = lymph stagnation, spleen stress
  - Center crack = digestion issues
  - Yellow = stressed liver
  - White coating = yeast overload
  - Strawberry burns = check PH for acidity
  - Inflamed = check iron
  - Painful or burning = check vitamin B-2

Muscles

- Weak contraction = not digesting carbs, check potassium
- Weak or slow reflex = check potassium
- Cannot relax muscles = check calcium, magnesium, sodium, water intake
- Lacking coordination or balance = check manganese
- Cramps at night = not digesting proteins, check calcium, magnesium
- Cramps during exercise = not digesting carbs, check calcium, magnesium
- Degeneration = check sodium
- Pain around joints = yeast overload, check sugar intake
- Tone deficient = check magnesium, vitamin D
- Fatigue quickly, but recover quickly = check circulation
- Shoulder tension (difficulty raising arms above head) = not digesting fats

Nails

- General poor condition = check selenium
- Dry = check vitamin F
- Fungus = yeast overload, probiotics
- Vertical grooves = not absorbing nutrients, so check small intestine, yeast overload, need of enzymes
- Horizontal grooves = adrenal stress
- Dark lines or grooves = metal toxicity
- Nail bed turns white when fingers straight = check iron
- White spots that grow out = adrenal stress, check vitamin C, B-5
- White or opaque spots that don't grow out = check zinc

- Hooked shape = respiratory stress
- Thickened = yeast overload, probiotics
- Splitting horizontally = check calcium
- Clear instead of white at ends = check calcium
- Length less than width = check heart
- Cuticle on thumb is pointed = check heart
- Red in corners of moon = lacking oxygen
- Pointed moon shape = check iodine, hypothyroid
- Moon on small finger = check heart and circulation
- Small or no moon on thumb = check calcium
- Moons showing on only 1 hand = check heart

Neck

- Creases across, middle and just below neck = check iodine, thyroid
- Enlarged thyroid area = check iodine, thyroid

Nerves

- General issues = check magnesium, vitamin B-12
- Pain = check calcium, magnesium
- Electrical sensations = check calcium, and excess iron

Nose

- Frequent nose bleeds = check vitamin C, water intake
- Sinus drip (chronic) = check iodine
- Loss of smell = check zinc
- Bulbous tip = check heart and circulation
- Cleft on tip = stronger indicator of heart and circulation
- Dry = not digesting carbs

Reproduction

- General challenges = check vitamin E, fat digestion
- Fertility issues = check manganese, vitamin A, not digesting fats
- Low sperm count = check selenium, not digesting fats
- Hot flashes = check vitamin F, not digesting fats
- Cramps = not digesting proteins
- Menstrual problems = check yeast overload
- Heavy = check vitamin C
- Scanty or absent = check vitamin F, extreme exercise
- Miscarriage = not digesting fats, check iodine (thyroid)
- Cannot induce labor = not digesting fats
- PMS = check vitamin E
- Postpartum depression = check for excess copper
- Prostate gland = general = not digesting protein, check lycopene, vitamin F
- Inflammation = check copper, zinc

Shoulders

- Pain in non-dominant shoulder = check vitamin B-12
- Raised towards ears = check vitamin C, B-5
- Rounded forward = check iodine, thyroid
- Can't raise arms above head, or trap muscles sore = not digesting fats
- Top edge of shoulder joint tender = check vitamin B-12

Skin / tissue

- Bed sores = check copper
- Bruise easily = check vitamin C, spleen
- Calcification of soft tissue = check for excess calcium and low phosphorous

- Lacking collagen = check vitamin C, not digesting proteins
- Dehydrated = water intake, not digesting carbs
- Weak connective tissue (sprains easily) = check manganese
- Dry, itchy, hives rash = probiotics and yeast overgrowth
- Dry, rough = check vitamin F, water intake, digesting fats
- Dry, dandruff, boils = not digesting of fats
- Dry, scaly, goose-bump like bumps = check vitamin A
- Orifice tissue is poor quality = check vitamin A
- Pale color for your skin type = check iron
- Naturally very fair or dark = melatonin needs are different check copper
- Psoriasis = check chromium, vitamin D
- Does not repair quickly (slow healing) = not digesting proteins, vitamin C
- Sensitive to sun = check copper
- Excessive sweating = check trace minerals
- Swelling, or retaining water = not digesting proteins, leaky gut

Urinary system

- Incontinence = probiotics, yeast overload
- Frequent infections = probiotics, yeast overload
- Frequent urination = drinking large amounts of water all at once
- Dark, concentrated, or strong smelling urine = not enough water intake
- Kidney Stones = check vitamin C, not digesting fats
  - If from calcium oxalate = also check magnesium
- Diagnosed kidney function problems = check magnesium, vitamin B-5

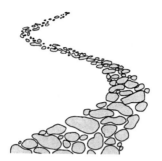

Reference: Recommended Books

I learned a great deal from these books. Their reference numbers throughout **Getting There** indicate they contain further information about that subject. I recommend making them part of your library. Enjoy them all!

(1) *Acupuncture Points, Images & Functions,* Arnie Lade
Specific information about each acupoint.

(2) *The Amazing Power of Deliberate Intent,* Esther and Jerry Hicks
The teachings of Abraham for using intent to create your life.

(3) The Anatomy of Stretching, Brad Walker
Illustrated guide for flexibility and injury rehabilitation.

(4) *Animal Speak,* Ted Andrews
What message are the animals giving you.

(5) *The Biology of Belief* and *Nature and Nurture,* Bruce Lipton, Ph.D. brucelipton.com, books/videos/youtube
How beliefs influence DNA and change our cells.

(6) *The Compete Dictionary of Ailments and Diseases,* Jacques Martel
A comprehensive list of where emotions are stored in the body

(7) *The Crystal Bible,* Judy Hall
A guide to crystals and what their frequencies can be used for.

(8) *Eat Fat, Get Thin,* Mark Hyman, M.D., Functional medicine, books/videos
Eating for your health.

(9) *The Enzyme Advantage: for Health Care Providers and People Who Care About Their Health,* Dr. Howard R. Loomis Jr., books and classes, foodenzymeinstitute.com
About digestion and enzymes and why you need them.

(10) *The Essential Book of Traditional Chinese Medicine,* Liu Yanchi
For the theories behind acupressure/acupuncture.

(11) *Essential Oils Desk Reference,* Life Science Publishing
A guide to essential oils and their uses.

(12) *Excuse Me, Your Life is Waiting,* Lynn Grabhorn
The "law of attraction" and how you can use it to your benefit.

(13) *The Field,* Lynne McTaggert
For science discoveries about the universal energy field and how we are all connected.

(14) *Functionalmedicine.org,* articles/videos
Information about functional medicine and practitioner locator

(15) *Hands of Light,* Barbara Ann Brennan
All about the human energy field

(16) *Messages from Water* and *The Hidden Messages in Water,* Masaru Emoto
The power of the written word to change water, and therefore us.

(17) *Molecules of Emotion,* Candace Pert, Ph.D.
How emotions are stored in cells and about the science research empire.

(18) *A New Earth,* Eckhart Tolle
How to live your life in order to create a new you and new world.

(19) *Path of Empowerment,* Barbara Marciniak, books/CDs/ newsletter, pleiadians.com
Wisdom for a World in Chaos.

(20) *The Power of Intention,* Wayne Dyer
Learning to Co-create Your World Your Way.

(21) *Recovery from Parkinson's* and *Once Upon a Pill* and *Medications of Parkinson's Disease,* Dr. Janice Walton-Hadlock, pdrecovery.org
An acupuncture study about curing PD.

(22) *The Secret,* Rhonda Byrne, books/videos/DVDs
How to use positive thinking and intention to expand your life.

(23) *Suckered,* Jeffrey Eisenberg, MD
All about sugar and how it affects our health.

(24) *Tapping Solutions,* Nick Ortner, thetappingsolution.com
How to use tapping on meridians to release old beliefs and create new.

(25) *What the Bleep Do We Know,* a movie DVD, whatthebleep.com
The link between emotions and our habits and reactions

(26) *You Can Heal Your Life,* Louise Hay
Emotional influence on the body and introduction to where they are stored

(27) *You Take Too Big a Bite,* Dr. Louis De Palma
About digestion and eating the proper foods, for kids of all ages.

Books not referenced, but interesting reads that pertain to *Getting There:*

Acu-Dog and *Acu-Cat* and *Acu-Horse,* Nancy Zidonis and Amy Snow, books/classes/on-line courses/charts, animalacupressure.com
Acupressure you can apply yourself to help your pets (and you). Their on-line classes make it simple.

Betrayal—The Series, Dr. Tom O'Bryan, A video series (betrayalseries.com)
Revealing the betrayal about autoimmune diseases and what you can do to help yourself.

Coyote Medicine, Lewis Mehl-Madrona, M.D.
How the AMA indoctrinates its new members.

Creating True Peace, Thich Nhat Hanh
Practices for creating peace for all aspects of life.

The Creation of Health, Carolyn Myss, Ph.D. and C. Norman Shealy, M.D.
About emotional responses that promote health

Einstein's Moon, F. David Peat
Explanation of energy effects at a distance.

The Emerging Mind, Karen N. Shanor, Ph.D.
The power of the mind.

Four Paws Five Directions, Cheryl Schwartz, DVM
Acupressure and Chinese medicine guide for your dogs and cats.

I Dare You!, William Danforth
For motivating yourself and others into making positive changes.

Inside Out, A Disney Pixar Movie
Cartoon movie about emotions for kids of all ages.

Learned Optimism, Martin Seligman
Power of positive thinking.

Mutant Message Down Under, Marlo Morgan
A journey with the Aborigines telling of their cooperative and connected lives.

No Grain, No Pain, Peter Osborne
A diet to ease chronic pain

The Oneness of Being, Dr. Marilyn Gewacke
Going in depth about healing the self and manifesting the soul's potential.

Who's Afraid Of Schrodinger's Cat? Ian Marshall and Danah Zohar
For explanations of the "new" sciences, such as chaos theory, quantum mechanics, neutrinos, wormholes, and models of the mind.

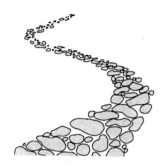

About the Author

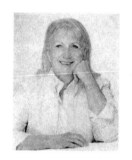

Jean Bennett is a holistic health care practitioner. In short, *she assists people in getting and staying well, specializing in chronic issues.* She helps people who have been everywhere and done everything to get rid of their pain, but have found no answers.

Jean's unique set of skills gives her a visionary perspective and a tenacity to see through the many messages the body is continuously conveying to us, and translate them into a plan for wellness. She has expertly blended her life's experience, formal training (acupressure, energy therapy, massage, and digestion) and her inborn skills (intuition, patience, logic, compassion, and persistence). This allowed her to become the expert in her field of healing the body through listening to it and providing what it needs.

She views herself as an educator who is passing on information that has not been part of our societal upbringing: *We can heal ourselves if we know how and are willing to do the work.* She has taken on the mission of helping people understand how to listen to their bodies, translate the messages, and navigate holistic care, so they can accomplish the full splendor of their lives.

Check out her website, www.jeanbennett.net for updated information about **Getting There**. You may also be interested in the "Body Babble Analysis" that helps track your changes from year to year. Your comments are welcome. Please email them to jean@jeanbennett.net or mail to PO Box 660, Webster, NY 14580.

CPSIA information can be obtained
at www.ICGtesting.com
Printed in the USA
FFOW01n0435170117
31430FF